first place
4 health
Bible Study Series

fit & healthy
summer

Lucinda Secrest McDowell

Published by Gospel Light
Ventura, California, U.S.A.
www.gospellight.com
Printed in the U.S.A.

Caution: The information contained in this book is intended to be solely for
informational and educational purposes. It is assumed that the First Place 4 Health
participant will consult a medical or health professional before beginning this or
any other weight-loss or physical fitness program.

Library of Congress Cataloging-in-Publication Data
McDowell, Lucinda Secrest, 1953-
Fit and healthy summer / Lucinda Secrest McDowell.
p. cm. — (First place 4 health summer Bible study)
ISBN 978-0-8307-5516-5 (trade paper)
1. Health—Religious aspects—Christianity—Textbooks. 2. Spiritual life—
Christianity—Textbooks. 3. Spiritual life—Biblical teaching. I. Title.
BT732.M33 2010
220.8′61304244—dc22
2010043021

Rights for publishing this book outside the U.S.A. or in non-English
languages are administered by Gospel Light Worldwide, an international
not-for-profit ministry. For additional information, please visit
www.glww.org, email info@glww.org, or write to Gospel Light Worldwide,
1957 Eastman Avenue, Ventura, CA 93003, U.S.A.

To order copies of this book and other Gospel Light products in bulk
quantities, please contact us at 1-800-446-7735.

contents

about the author

Lucinda Secrest McDowell, a graduate of Gordon-Conwell Theological Seminary, is an international conference speaker and author of nine books, including the First Place 4 Health Bible Study *God's Purpose for You* and *30 Ways to Embrace Life, Spa for the Soul, Amazed by Grace* and *Role of a Lifetime*. She has also written for 50 magazines and been a contributing author to 25 other books. A wife and mother of four, Cindy writes and speaks from New England through her ministry Encouraging Words that Transform. She leads a First Place 4 Health class for women and men in the Hartford area and is also part of a First Place 4 Health authors group, helping to coordinate their annual wellness week. Visit Cindy's website at **www.EncouragingWords.net** or contact her at **cindy@encouragingwords.net**.

introduction

But seek first his kingdom and his righteousness,
and all these things will be given to you as well.
MATTHEW 6:33

Summertime can be filled with trips, summer camps and other disruptions in schedules that make it difficult to remain faithful to your commitment to living healthy. *Healthy Summer Living* is a six-week study that was written to provide order to you during the busy summer season without being a burden on your time. It will give you inspiration for each day and also challenge you to stay on course by applying the truths at the core of First Place 4 Health.

You can do this study on your own, or as part of a family devotion time in the home, or in conjunction with a special summer First Place 4 Health group. The Bible study has been created in a five-day format, with the last two days reserved for reflection on the material studied. Keep in mind that the ultimate goal of studying the Bible is not only for knowledge but also for application and a changed life.

Don't feel anxious if you can't seem to find the *correct* answer. Many times, the Word will speak differently to different people, depending on where they are in their walk with God and the season of life they are experiencing. If you are doing this study as part of a special summer group, be prepared to discuss with your fellow members what you learned that week through your study.

There are some additional components included with this study that will be helpful as you pursue the goal of giving Christ first place in every area of your life:

- **Group Prayer Request Form:** This form is at the end of each week's study. If you are using this study as part of a group, you can record any special requests that might be given in class.

- **Summertime Helps:** These are valuable tips and suggestions for staying healthy spiritually, mentally, emotionally and physically throughout the summer season.

- **Leader Discussion Guide:** This discussion guide is provided to help the First Place 4 Health leader guide a group through this Bible study. It includes ideas for facilitating a First Place 4 Health class discussion for each week of the Bible study.

- **Two Weeks of Menu Plans with Recipes:** There are 14 days of meals, and each of the days are interchangeable. Each day totals 1,400 to 1,500 calories and includes snacks. Instructions are given for those who need more calories, and recipes for additional summer favorites are included with the menus. An accompanying grocery list includes items that will be needed for each week of meals.

- **First Place 4 Health Member Survey:** If you are using this study as part of a group, fill out this survey and bring it to your first meeting. This information will help your leader know your interests and talents.

- **Personal Weight and Measurement Record:** Use this form to keep a record of your weight loss during the six weeks of the study.

- **Weekly Prayer Partner Forms:** If you are attending a summer session of First Place 4 Health, fill out the weekly prayer partner form and put it into a basket during the meeting. After the meeting, you will draw out a prayer request form, and this will be your prayer partner for the week.

- **Live It Trackers:** The Live It Tracker is for you to complete at home and turn in to your leader at your weekly meetings. If you have a plan, you can remain consistent in practicing the spiritual, mental, emotional and physical disciplines you have begun in First Place 4 Health—even through the summer!

- **Scripture Memory Cards:** These cards have been designed so that you can use them while exercising. It is suggested that you punch a hole in the upper left corner and place the cards on a ring. You may want to take the cards in the car or to work so that you can practice each week's Scripture memory verse throughout the day.

Before you begin your first week of this study, take a moment to write down your goals and strategies for this summer as they pertain to maintaining your spiritual, mental, emotional and physical health.

My goals for this summer are:

Spiritual: _____

_____

_____

_____

_____

_____

Mental: _____

_____

_____

_____

_____

Emotional: _____

_____

_____

_____

_____

_____

_____

Physical: _____

_____

_____

_____

_____

_____

_____

My strategies for reaching those goals are:

Spiritual: _____

_____

_____

_____

_____

_____

Mental: _____

_____

_____

_____

_____

_____

_____

Emotional: _____

_____

_____

_____

_____

_____

_____

Physical: _____

_____

_____

_____

_____

_____

May the next six weeks take you on a joyful journey toward complete wholeness and health! Here's to the journey!

maps

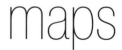

SCRIPTURE MEMORY VERSE
I will instruct you and teach you in the way you should go;
I will counsel you and watch over you.
PSALM 32:8

Helpful websites such as MapQuest or Google Maps are wonderful for offering explicit instructions to help get you from point A to point B (presumably in the quickest and most direct route). All you have to do is enter where you want to start and where you want to end and you have a step-by-step set of instructions including every twist and turn along the way.

Do you ever wish there was a map website for life's journey? So there would never be any doubt as to whether to turn left or right? So you could clearly see ahead the rocky roads and unexpected detours? So you would know how to pack for any contingency? So you would be assured that you're headed toward the right destination?

Yes, it would be nice to have a complete set of instructions that warned of problem areas, but that would eliminate the need for faith and trust in God as we journey on to each next step. We are all somewhere on that faith journey—some just starting out, others well along the way, and still others in the process of navigating back on track from significant detours.

Our faith journey is similar in concept to our journey toward balanced health physically, mentally, spiritually and emotionally. This process is indeed a journey, but it's more like taking "the long way" instead of the quickest route. Changing old habits and replacing them with a healthier lifestyle takes time and occurs over several seasons.

Summer can be a significant time for either jump-starting or recharging our health pursuits. At first glance, the weather, vacation plans and other seasonal variables seem to make this season conducive for such pursuits. However, most of us have learned that very few things in life happen automatically. We have to intentionally decide to live a life of faith, as well as to make this summer's journey a fit and healthy one.

Fortunately, as we seek God's wisdom and guidance on moving forward in our journey of faith, this week's memory verse reminds us that God will always be with us on our journey. Indeed, He is willing and able to not only show us the way to go, but also to travel alongside us.

Day 1

DIRECTIONS

Dear heavenly Father, I'm off on a new journey, and I desperately need You to guide me in the right direction. Thank You for promising to show me the best way to a life that honors You. Amen.

When preparing to travel somewhere you've never been, where do you go for directions? Do you visit an Internet website? Do you consult a GPS? Do you ask a friend who has been there before? Do you ever wonder about the reliability of your source of information?

Read Psalm 25:4-10. In verses 4-5, what three things does the psalmist ask God to provide?

1. _____

_____

2. _____

_____

3. _____

_____

According to verses 6-7, what does the psalmist ask God to remember? What does the psalmist ask God to forget?

_____

_____

_____

_____

_____

_____

In the book *God's Road Map for Women,* David Bordon and Thomas Winters have the following to say about how to know whether you're following God's directions:

> As with any journey you take, it's vitally important to first make sure you're headed in the right direction. So, each morning, check out your landmarks. Look for direction and insight by reading God's words in the Bible. Take a few moments to talk to God in prayer. Look back over where you traveled the day before and talk with God about anything you wish you'd done differently. Ask Him to help lead you today to make decisions that will draw you closer to Him. Then, venture out into the world with confidence. God has the itinerary for your life held firmly in His hand. Today is yet one more step on the journey He has planned for you to take together—an adventure that will last throughout eternity.[1]

According to verses 8-10, why is God reliable—why is the psalmist sure that God will indeed provide direction for his journey (and ours)?

_____

_____

_____

_____

_____

Read Psalm 119:9-11. What guides us on our journey—what lights our path?

_____

_____

_____

_____

How do we keep from straying from God's directions for our journey—how do we stay on the path?

_____

_____

_____

_____

O Lord, Your Word is true and timely for me today. Help me to know You better by studying Your precepts and directions in Scripture. Thank You for helping me in the process. Amen.

Day 2 DEPENDENCE

Dear God, You know and I know that I cannot make any substantial changes in my life without Your help. May I always seek You first and consult You each step of the way. Amen.

In many parts of the Bible, agrarian imagery was used to clearly communicate to people who lived off the land. Read Hosea 10:12-13. Rewrite in your own words the phrases in verse 12.

"Sow for yourselves righteousness"

_____

_____

_____

"Reap the fruit of unfailing love"

_____
_____
_____
_____

"Break up your unplowed ground"

_____
_____
_____
_____

"Seek the LORD until he comes"

_____
_____
_____
_____

What "unplowed ground" is there in your life? What parts of your life have become hardened by neglect?

_____
_____
_____
_____
_____

In what specific ways can you "break up" the hardened areas in your life?

_____
_____
_____
_____
_____

One of the reasons people sometimes fail in healthy and in godly pursuits is that they depend totally on their own willpower. According to verse 13, what are the three consequences of depending on your own strength?

1. _____

2. _____

3. _____

How will you depend on God and His Map on your summer quest?

_____

_____

_____

_____

_____

_____

In *Fathered by God,* John Eldredge states the following:

> The pleasure of a map is that it gives you the lay of the land, and yet you still have to make choices about how you will cover the terrain before you. A map is a guide, not a formula. It offers freedom. It does not tell you how fast to walk, though when you see the contour lines growing very close together, you know you are approaching steep terrain and will want to mend your stride. It does not tell you why the mountain is there, or how old the forest is. It tells you how to get where you are going.[2]

It is only God on whom we can depend for the "living water," the eternal life, which is the ultimate goal of our journey (see John 4:10).

> *Lord, make me willing to follow where You lead, and help me to depend only on You and Your Word for the direction I should go. Amen.*

DISCIPLINE

*Dear God, I don't know why it is so hard for me to do the right
thing every time. But I do desire to live a disciplined life, and I thank
You that You will help me make good choices. Amen.*

Psalm 119, the longest psalm in the Bible, is all about God's laws, precepts, statutes and decrees. What do the words "law," "precept," "statute"
and "decree" mean?

_____

_____

_____

_____

Read Psalm 119:105-112. How does God's Word light the path (see verse
105)?

_____

_____

_____

_____

According to verse 106, what is the only way we can travel the true path
for which God provides light?

_____

_____

_____

_____

What "snares" have you encountered (see verse 110)? Who or what has
tried to make you turn away from following God's Word?

_____

_____

_____

_____

What should keep you disciplined so that you can avoid those challenges or snares?

_____

_____

_____

_____

_____

Exercise is one area that can be particularly hard for some people to be disciplined about in their First Place 4 Health journey. What specific tools or strategies help you not to stray from your exercise plan? (For example, have you joined a class, do you write reminders on your calendar, or do you exercise with a partner?)

_____

_____

_____

_____

_____

Dr. Edmund A. Taub says, "Perhaps the most important benefit [of exercise] is the effect it has on your psychological and spiritual outlook. When you feel better about yourself, when you feel empowered and energetic, you make healthier choices in your eating and life-style habits.[3] Exercise can lift your spirits, but according to verses 111-112, what brings true joy to the human heart, and how is that joy sustained?

_____

_____

_____

_____

_____

O Lord, I do commit my life journey into Your hands, and I ask that
You give me the strength and discipline I need to stay the course. Amen.

DISCERNMENT

*Gracious and loving God, I'm so grateful to be in this study and
on this journey, but I need help in discerning the right choices
each time I come to a crossroads on my journey. May I trust You,
because I know that You are indeed trustworthy. Amen.*

On our faith journey, it is important to walk in partnership with God as
our ultimate guide. Read Proverbs 16:9. How does the partnership between God and us work?

_____

_____

_____

_____

_____

We can plan and dream and even scheme all we want, but it is God who
will actually decide where we will go and what our journey will be. Mary
Beth Chapman discovered this, and in her autobiography, *Learning to
See: A Journey of Struggle and Hope,* she tells about how God's journey for
her wasn't at all what she had planned or expected:

> As long as I can remember . . . I've held on to certain expecta-
> tions about life. But Jesus has always loved me enough to show
> me that even when I push my own ideas and expectations, He is
> there to guide me back to green pastures. He has shepherded me
> through the mountainous terrain of my stubbornness, shame,
> depression, and inadequacy and brought me gently back to the
> lushness of His love. He loves us enough to never let us go . . .
> even when it feels like He has.
>
> It wasn't like I wanted a life that was unreasonable or ques-
> tionable. My plans had to do with a Christ-centered ministry, an
> easy marriage, a peaceful and orderly home, constructive growth
> rather than shattered dreams, protection rather than fires . . . all

good things. Still, God has turned my life, my expectations, and some of my dreams completely upside down so many times.

In the midst of the journey, God really is with us and for us. I have found that even during those times when the path is darkest, He leaves little bits of evidence all along the way—that can give me what I need to take the next step. But I can only find them if I choose to SEE.[4]

According to the dictionary, "discernment" means "the quality of being able to grasp and comprehend what is obscure."[5] How amazing that God offers us this ability! Read Proverbs 2:6-8. What are the seven gifts/actions God provides to us?

1. _____
2. _____
3. _____
4. _____
5. _____
6. _____
7. _____

Which of these gifts are you most in need of in order to discern God's leading in your life? Why?

_____
_____
_____
_____
_____
_____

Dear God, thank You for providing me with discernment so that I can see the way that I should go. Help me not to veer to the right or to the left of Your leading, and please continue to guard my way. Amen.

DEDICATION

Dear heavenly Father, I dedicate all my efforts to You. I pray that I might live a holy life and make choices that are pleasing to You and beneficial for my body and soul. Amen.

When we dedicate, or devote, ourselves to God and His ways, God will help us along our journey. Read Proverbs 3:5-6. When we commit ourselves to serve God whole-heartedly, what will God do?

_____

_____

_____

_____

Read Psalm 17:5-8. As we journey together with God, what are we to do? What will God do?

My part	God's part
When I . . .	He . . .
When I . . .	He . . .
When I . . .	He . . .
When I . . .	He . . .

Read Psalm 1:1-2. As we continue our walk with God, what should we do "day and night"?

_____

_____

_____

_____

_____

By studying the Bible and memorizing Scripture, we show our commitment, our dedication, to God for our life's journey. When we start on a road trip, it wouldn't make sense for us to have a map in the glove compartment or GPS on the dashboard if we never consulted it.

God's Word is more than just another book on the shelf. It's a Road Map for life. Unlike a regular map that contains street names and mileage markers, this Map is written in love letters, history lessons, prophecies, proverbs, biographies, poetry—even postcards from the borders of heaven that sometimes sound like science fiction. But there is a thread of truth running through it all—truth that remains steadfast throughout centuries, millenniums, and eternity itself. This truth helps provide you with what you need to know to navigate your way through time toward heaven.[6]

Every day is unexplored territory. It's easy to get lost or sidetracked on the way. But the more familiar we are with God and His Map, the Bible, the easier we will be able to discern His hand along the way.

*God, make me continuously turn to Your Map—Your Word of truth—
for I know that without it I will continue to follow the next-best thing
instead of seek the ultimate prize. Amen.*

Day 6 REFLECTION AND APPLICATION

*Dear God, I hate to admit it, but I do have enemies who are not
supportive of this new path. Please give me strength and protection as I
continue toward You and my new spiritual and physical goals. Amen.*

Many of the psalms were written by King David, who experienced God's deliverance from a number of different enemies, including members of his own family. Read Psalm 16:8-11. According to verses 8-10, what was the source of David's ability to "not be shaken" and to "rest secure?"

_____

_____

_____

_____

What "enemies" do you have to battle as you seek balanced health? From what and/or whom do you need God to deliver you?

_____

_____

_____

_____

Do you believe God will guide and provide direction in your life? What three promises in verse 11 are true for the both the psalmist and us?

1. _____

2. _____

3. _____

Thank You, King of kings, for being my deliverer and my shield when I need a strong arm and a serious ally. May I not be shaken or stressed when challenges come my way, because You are here with me. Amen.

REFLECTION AND APPLICATION

Day **7**

Almighty God, I still have a hard time understanding that Your love for me is endless and unconditional. But I pray that I might live as Your beloved and give You cause for much delight. Amen.

Our heavenly Father not only wants to show us His way from start to finish, but He also wants to shower His love and care upon us in the process. Read Psalm 37:23-24. Our Lord both delights in us and upholds us on the path. It's true! Now imagine God speaking to you today. Fill in what He might say.

"I delight in your . . .

_____

_____

_____

_____

_____

"I want to uphold you when . . .

_____

_____

_____

_____

_____

. . . because I love you." Your heavenly Father.

Singer Natalie Grant once found herself totally overwhelmed in discovering that God actually delighted in her:

> I cannot begin to tell you how freeing it was when I first embraced Jesus Christ as my real Friend. . . . I had always been told of God's great love, and somewhere inside I believed it. But what completely melted my heart, what completely liberated me from choking insecurity, wasn't just the truth that Jesus loved me but that Jesus liked me—but that Jesus LIKED me! Exactly as I was. I didn't have to pretend: I didn't have to be a certain size or wear the right jeans. I could be having a bad-hair day, and He would still like me.[7]

As we conclude this week's study, read Jeremiah 29:11-13. According to verse 11, what two gifts does God promise you?

1. _____

2. _____

In verses 12-13, what four things are you to do as a result of moving forward into that future?

1. _____

2. _____

3. _____

4. _____

Jesus, lover of my soul, thank You for loving me as I am and for loving me too much to leave me here. Take my life and make me a willing servant of Yours, a worshiping child who follows Your plan and purpose for my life.

Notes

1. David Bordon and Thomas J. Winters, *God's Road Map for Women* (Tulsa, OK: Bordon-Winters, 2006), p. 45.
2. John Eldredge, *Fathered by God* (Nashville, TN: Thomas Nelson Publishers, 2009), p. xi.
3. Edward A. Taub, *Balance Your Body, Balance Your Life: Total Health Rejuvenation* (New York: Pocket Books, 1999), p. 335.
4. Mary Beth Chapman, *Learning to See: A Journey of Struggle and Hope* (Grand Rapids, MI: Revell, 2010), p. 26.
5. *Merriam-Webster's Collegiate Dictionary*, 11th ed., s.v. "discernment."
6. Bordon and Winters, *God's Road Map for Women*, p. 93.
7. Natalie Grant, *The Real Me: Being the Girl God Sees* (Nashville, TN: W Publishing Group, 2005), p. 91.

Group Prayer Requests

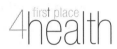

Today's Date: _____

Name	Request

Results

_____

_____

_____

_____

_____

baggage

SCRIPTURE MEMORY VERSE
*Praise be to the Lord, to God our Savior,
who daily bears our burdens.*
PSALM 68:19

Are you one of those travelers who take everything but the kitchen sink when you go on a trip? Well, if your journey includes air travel, be prepared to pay for that privilege! These days, checking luggage for flights can be expensive.

Most carriers only allow a free carry-on bag and a briefcase or a purse for each passenger. But even those items can be hard to stow overhead if you're one of the last to board the plane. Friends, it's time to unpack the "stuff" and learn to travel lightly.

Everyone has baggage from life's journey, and, quite frankly, these burdens often demand a price from us that gets harder and harder to pay. We find that lugging all that old junk around keeps us from freely moving forward. Do you want to unload some "stuff" this summer? Hey, it's a grand time for coming clean and starting fresh!

The best part of all is that God wants us to give all our baggage— all our burdens that we have been carrying—to Him and to let Him carry them for us. This week's memory verse in Psalm 68:19 reminds us to thank Him each day for this faith-journey perk, which doesn't even come with an add-on fee.

But first, let's examine our baggage cart and start eliminating the extra weight.

FLESH

*God, my Father, please help me when I am tempted to give in to what
I want and to things that bring instant gratification. Amen.*

Read 1 Thessalonians 4:3-7. What does being "sanctified" and "live a
holy life" mean (verses 3,7)?

_____

_____

_____

_____

According to verse 4, what is the key to fighting the temptation to give
in to fleshly desires?

_____

_____

_____

_____

Read 2 Samuel 11:1-5. This passage begins the sad story of a time when
King David gave in to his fleshly desires. The story starts with a de-
scription of the season: "in the spring, at the time when kings go off to
war." But what did King David do (see verse 1)?

_____

_____

_____

_____

What happened as a result of David's not doing what he was supposed
to be doing (see verses 2-5)?

_____

_____

_____

_____

In what ways have you given in to the demands of your flesh, even as you know you want to seek balanced health?

_____

_____

_____

_____

_____

What potential consequences lie ahead if you continue on that path?

_____

_____

_____

_____

_____

In what specific ways can you combat desires of the flesh?

_____

_____

_____

O Lord, I want to spend each moment of each day doing
exactly what You have called me to do. Help me not to give in to
desires of the flesh but to stay on track. Amen.

FAILURE

Day 2

Most merciful God, I know what it is to have failed You and
hurt others in the process. May I learn hard lessons from those times
so that I may go forth into a future of hope and mercy. Amen.

Read 2 Samuel 11:6-17,26-27. These passages continue the story of King David's moral failure as his sins began to mount up to include not only adultery but also murder. According to verses 6-8, how did David connive to keep his infidelity and parentage of Bathsheba's baby a secret?

_____

_____

_____

_____

_____

_____

In verses 9-13, how did Uriah inadvertently thwart David's sneaky plans?

_____

_____

_____

_____

_____

According to verses 14-17, what extreme measure did David take in order to cover up his sin?

_____

_____

_____

_____

_____

David ended up marrying Bathsheba, but who was most "displeased" by David and Bathsheba's failure to obey God's commands (see verse 27)?

_____

_____

_____

_____

Our sins have the same result. How do you feel when you know that you have failed to obey God's commands or displeased the Lord?

_____

_____

_____

_____

_____

What specifically have you done (or can you do) to make clear to God that you're sorry for any past failures and that you want to do better?

_____

_____

_____

_____

O Lord, I know that I have failed sometimes to obey Your commands. I want to always return to Your ways and the path that You have laid out for me. Amen.

FACE THE FACTS   Day 3

Gracious and loving God, I am glad that You sometimes force me to face hard facts about myself and my actions. Thank You for times when You have pointed out my rebellion to me and then offered me another chance. Amen.

Just as David and Bathsheba had to face the fact that the sins they carried weighed them down, our own sins weigh on us, and we end up carrying far too much baggage. Jen Hatmaker, Christian author and speaker, describes how to handle this baggage:

Here's the truth: You can't really travel this road when you're loaded down with sin. You may carry so much sinful baggage, you've literally come to a screeching halt. Or you may manage to move slowly, but carrying your sin is like pulling a trailer. Everyone is passing you, and the slightest breeze sends you all over the road. Either way, Jesus wants you to feel the wind in your hair, and sin can only hinder your progress. This includes sin in action, motive or thought.[1]

In other words, we need to face the fact of our sins before we can deal with them and be free to move along on our journey. The conclusion of the story of David and Bathsheba is told in 2 Samuel 12. Read verses 1-14. Like many of us, David was either unable or unwilling to see his own sin. What clever way did the prophet Nathan use to force his king to face facts?

_____

_____

_____

_____

_____

When the light finally dawned for David, what did he say (see verse 13)?

_____

_____

_____

_____

_____

Just because we confess our sins and receive forgiveness from God does not mean that there won't be any consequences for our wrong actions. What happened as a consequence of David's sins (see verse 14)?

_____

_____

_____

_____

Facing the facts of our sins is a good first step to unpacking all the extra baggage we've been toting. In his book *Traveling Light,* minister and bestselling Christian author Max Lucado offers us extra-baggage handlers hope:

> God has a great race for you to run. Under His care you will go where you've never been and serve in ways you've never dreamed. But you have to drop some stuff. How can you share grace if you are full of guilt? How can you offer comfort if you are disheartened? How can you lift someone else's load if your arms are full with your own?
>
> For the sake of those you love, travel light.
>
> For the sake of the God you serve, travel light.
>
> For the sake of your own joy, travel light.
>
> There are certain weights in life you simply cannot carry. Your Lord is asking you to set them down and trust Him. He is the father at the baggage claim. When a dad sees his five-year-old son trying to drag the family trunk off the carousel, what does he say? The father will say to his son what God is saying to you.
>
> "Set it down, child. I'll carry that one."[2]

What are some of the burdens you need to let go of so God can carry them for you?

_____

_____

_____

_____

_____

Father God, I'm so glad that You really are willing to take these burdens from me. This extra baggage has weighed me down and slowed my journey. Today, I gladly place it into Your hands. Amen.

FORGIVEN

*Jesus, You are the One who died so that my sins would be forgiven. How can I
ever thank You? I come to You today with a humble heart, asking that once
again You make me clean and launch me on Your straight path. Amen.*

Even though a major impediment on our walk of faith is the weight of
sinful baggage, we can receive a major boost when we confess our sins
and receive God's forgiveness. How fortunate we are that God's Word
not only contains the story you've studied the past few days but also a
beautiful record of King David's own time with God.

Read Psalm 51:1-17. What are the four things David entreated God to do
(see verses 1-2)?

1. _____

2. _____

3. _____

4. _____

How will you depend on God and His Map on your summer quest?

_____
_____
_____
_____

According to verse 6, God desires "truth in the inner parts." How did
David confess the truth to Him in verses 3-5?

_____
_____
_____
_____
_____

David continues in verses 7-15 to beseech God for cleansing, healing and help. What does David want God to do for him (see verses 10-12)?

_____

_____

_____

_____

According to verses 13-16, what does David plan to do once God forgives him?

_____

_____

_____

_____

In your own words, what does God want us to offer Him (see verse 17)?

_____

_____

_____

_____

It's unfortunate that even though God does forgive us when we confess our sins, sometimes we have trouble accepting God's forgiveness, and we continue to be burdened by our guilt for committing the sin in the first place. Christian author and speaker Nancie Carmichael discusses this burden of guilt in her book _Surviving One Bad Year: 7 Spiritual Strategies to Lead You to a New Beginning_:

> Guilt, anger, and shame can be so deeply ingrained in our hearts that they color everything in our lives, and we're not even aware they are there. But they weigh us down and keep us from joyfully running the race God has set before us.
> When we are confronted by the ugly presence of these emotions, we must realize that the harsh voice of bitterness and

condemnation is not God's voice—it is the voice of the enemy of our soul, the accuser of God's children. And we must not agree with him. Even when we've made mistakes, if we have asked forgiveness from God and others for real or perceived failings, then we must let it go. Leave it. But often the last person we let off the hook is our own selves. . . .

We can spend a lot of time trying to fix what went wrong. But we cannot heal the deepest hurts. Only God can. And only we can allow Him to do it. Forgiveness is the only answer when we have no other answer.[3]

Recent medical research studies, such as the Stanford Forgiveness Project, have shown that forgiving others—and ourselves—is good for a person's health. Here are some of the physical benefits that people who forgive may enjoy:

- Up to 50 percent less stress and anxiety
- Better sleep
- Lowered risk of heart disease and heart attacks
- A stronger nervous system
- Lowered blood pressure
- Fewer headaches and stomach aches
- Improved circulation
- Less depression[4]

We must forgive ourselves and others as God has forgiven us. Choosing forgiveness may be one of the smartest decisions a person can make for improving quality of health!

Merciful Savior, even though I have received forgiveness from You, it is sometimes hard for me to forgive myself. Yet I know that I cannot move forward without coming clean and accepting the work You have done for me. Today, I accept Your gift of forgiveness with humility and gratitude. Amen.

FREEDOM Day 5

O Lord, how I long to be free from all this "stuff" that weighs on my heart and keeps me down as I attempt to keep moving forward on the journey with You! Thank You for being the One who frees me. Amen.

Have you ever tried to run while tied to a ball and chain? It's practically impossible to walk, much less run. And that's one reason a ball and chain was a great deterrent to convicts working on a chain gang. But it's not at all appropriate for God's children who are seeking to grow in faith and move forward into a life of freedom and balance.

Read Romans 6:15-23. This powerful explanation of what freedom from sin really means should resonate with everyone who has ever found himself or herself enslaved to sin, be it an unhealthy habit, a toxic relationship, or something else. We are slaves to whomever or whatever we obey. According to the apostle Paul, to experience true freedom, to what should we become slaves (see verse 18)?

_____

_____

_____

What popular cultural worldviews of how a person must look, act, speak, spend and behave in order to be successful can enslave a person?

_____

_____

_____

_____

In what ways can you feel enslaved by the expectations and/or opinions of others?

_____

_____

_____

_____

"Juneteenth" is the name of an annual celebration commemorating June 19, 1865, when Texas slaves learned that they were free. Technically, these slaves had been freed way back on January 1, 1863, when President Abraham Lincoln's Emancipation Proclamation first took effect, yet the African-Americans in Texas had continued living in slavery for more than two years! Unfortunately, many of us today are just like those freed slaves. Even though God has set us free from sin, we continue to live as slaves. However, God is the great emancipator! According to verses 22-23, what are the two results when you walk forward into that freedom?

1. _____

2. _____

As Charles Wesley once wrote, "My chains fell off! My heart was free! I rose, went forth, and followed Thee. Amazing love! How can it be? That Thou, my God, shouldst die for me?"[5]

Great God, my Emancipator, I am determined to live as a free person, no longer enslaved to the enemy of my soul or others who would have me believe lies. Thanks for Your amazing love that allows me to walk in new freedom today and always. Amen.

Day 6

REFLECTION AND APPLICATION

Dear God, You know how often I feel so alone, especially when it comes to trying to live a healthy and godly life. I know I cannot complete this journey all by myself. Thank You for remaining by my side and for bringing others alongside me. Amen.

In order to find greater balance in emotional health, First Place 4 Health emphasizes the importance of supporting one another in community.

God's people were never meant to journey alone, and we simply grow more and live healthier while in fellowship. Read Hebrews 3:12-14. What is the warning given here?

_____

_____

_____

_____

_____

_____

What is presented as a way to stay out of harm's way?

_____

_____

_____

_____

_____

In their book *God's Road Map for Women,* David Bordon and Thomas Winters tell us why fellowship ("roadside assistance") is so important:

> Everyone can use a little roadside assistance along the highway of life. At times, the journey can feel long. Certain stretches may seem lonely, monotonous, or dangerous. Some days may be uncomfortably bumpy, while others hold terrain that looks so unfamiliar you may fear you've lost your way. At times such as these, a little encouragement can go a long way: a note from a friend, a message on your voice mail that simply says "I love you," a hug when words aren't enough, a pat on the back from someone you look up to, an unexpected gift, a heartfelt smile, a timely word. When your heart needs a lift, lift up God's Word. You'll find these words of hope and healing have the power to lift your heart and your spirits, no matter how heavy they may be.[6]

What are some tangible ways you can encourage others on their faith journey?

_____

_____

_____

_____

Now put the name of a person you know next to each action. Pray that God will help you to encourage that person in that way sometime this week. Move beyond the praying—just do it! Now read Hebrews 3:14. According to this verse, what are we called to do?

_____

_____

_____

_____

In her book *Traveling Together*, Karla Worley offers the following practical advice on how we can encourage others:

> How can you, my friend in the faith, help me to become more like Christ? You can know me. You can be there. Hold me accountable for holy living. Encourage me to live the life of the Spirit. Model servanthood. Keep me active in worship and service. And you can do all this in the course of our days and years together, not just doing holy things, but understanding that all the things we do hold the possibility of the holy.[7]

Ecclesiastes 4:12 reminds us that "a cord of three strands is not quickly broken." So hold firmly to one another, and you will hold firmly to God.

Dearest Jesus, I want to be a faithful friend, and I pray that You will clearly show me how to reach out to others and give them some encouragement and support, even as I am refreshed by You. Amen.

REFLECTION AND APPLICATION

Faithful One, I cannot even begin to count all of the times and situations in which You have been faithful in relieving me of the burdens and encumbrances that would have held me back from receiving Your best. Today, I pray that I may respond to You in faith and fidelity. Amen.

Reflect on God's faithfulness in your life as you recall some of the unhealthy baggage that you have been traveling through life with so far. Now read Psalm 32:1-5. What are the characteristics of the person who is "blessed" (see verses 1-2)?

_____

_____

_____

_____

_____

_____

What happens to a person who does not put down their baggage and admit their sins (see verses 3-4)?

_____

_____

_____

_____

_____

According to verse 5, what is God faithful to do when a person confesses his or her sins?

_____

_____

_____

_____

_____

_____

How does this passage apply to your current situation?

_____

_____

_____

_____

_____

Perhaps today would be a great opportunity for you to take time in God's presence to unload your burdens and confess your sins. So, what baggage are you still carrying around on your journey? What is your heavy load? Think of it more as a backpack full of all your hurts, pain, unforgiveness and shattered dreams. When you carry that "stuff" around, it gets harder and harder to keep on walking.

As you conclude this week's session, imagine yourself sitting at the feet of Jesus and emptying out that backpack. Pause for a moment to symbolically take out each incident, each person, each time you were hurt or each time you inflicted hurt on someone else, and lay them at the feet of a loving Savior who has been longing to give you freedom.[8] Remember that God loves you and that He wants you to be free so that you can live the life He has intended for you!

My Lord, I am laying my sins at Your feet. You know that I cannot continue to carry this baggage anymore. It has already cost me way too much. Thank You that I can leave these burdens here with You and go my way free. Amen.

Notes

1. Jen Hatmaker, *Road Trip: Five Adventures You're Meant to Live: A Modern Girl's Bible Study* (Colorado Springs, CO: NavPress, 2006), p. 29.
2. Max Lucado, *Traveling Light: Releasing the Burdens You Were Never Intended to Bear* (Nashville, TN: Word Publishing, 2001), p. 8.
3. Nancie Carmichael, *Surviving One Bad Year: 7 Spiritual Strategies to Lead You to a New Beginning* (Nashville, TN: Howard Books, 2009).

4. A.H. Harris, F.M. Luskin, S.V. Benisovich, et al, "Effects of a Group Forgiveness Intervention on Forgiveness, Perceived Stress and Trait Anger: A Randomized Trial," *Journal of Clinical Psychology*, vol. 62, no. 6, pp. 715-733. http://learningtoforgive.com/research/effects-of-group-forgiveness-intervention-on-perceived-stress-state-and-trait-anger-symptoms-of-stress-self-reported-health-and-forgiveness-stanford-forgiveness-project/.

5. Charles Wesley (1707–1788), "And Can It Be That I Should Gain?" *Psalms and Hymns,* 1738.

6. David Bordon and Thomas J. Winters, *God's Road Map for Women*, (Tulsa, OK: Bordon-Winters, 2006), p. 53.

7. Karla Worley, *Traveling Together: Thoughts on Women, Friendship, and the Journey of Faith* (Birmingham, AL: New Hope Publishers, 2003), p. 43.

8. Lucinda Secrest McDowell, *Quilts from Heaven* (Nashville, TN: B & H Publishers, 2007), p. 126.

Group Prayer Requests

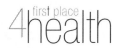

Today's Date: _____

Name	Request

Results

_____

_____

_____

_____

_____

new adventures

SCRIPTURE MEMORY VERSE
Blessed are those whose strength is in you,
who have set their hearts on pilgrimage.
PSALM 84:5

This summer, a young woman named Johanna went back to Baghdad—not once but twice. She traveled to that nation as part of a team to help rebuild that devastated country, but still her mother spent a lot of time praying for her protection. After all, this was the same gal who had to be evacuated from her West African Peace Corps village during a dangerous political uprising. Yet her mother knew that Johanna was a born adventurer. She had moved to a large European city to pursue her graduate degree and had traveled to India to set up women's microfinance projects. Truly, she was a young woman who had set her heart on pilgrimage and who found her strength in God.

What new adventures will you pursue this summer? How can you break out of your same-old, same-old and move forward into new dimensions of balanced health—spiritually, mentally, physically and emotionally? Have you asked God for the courage to take a risk for a new adventure?

In this week's memory verse, the word "pilgrimage," as you might expect, means the journey of a pilgrim. The word "pilgrim" comes from the Greek word *pareipidemos,* which simply means "people who spend their lives going someplace." That's what we are—Christ followers who spend our lives going to God. Perhaps we could join Augustine in praying the following:

I commit and commend myself unto You, in Whom I am and live, and know. Be the Goal of my pilgrimage, and my Rest by the way. Let my soul take refuge from the crowding turmoil of worldly thoughts beneath the shadow of Your wings; let my heart, this sea of restless waves, find peace in You O God. Amen.[1]

Our new adventure this summer *should* include a commitment (or a recommitment) to continue our faith journey with and to God.

Day 1

POSSIBILITIES

Dear God, I know there are great new possibilities for success this summer as I seek to maintain a balanced health regimen. I long to achieve my goals for this summer. I am ready for You to do a new thing in my life. Amen.

What "new thing" do you hope God will do in your life this summer?

_____
_____
_____
_____

What is your part in helping this to happen?

_____
_____
_____
_____

Read 1 Corinthians 2:9-10. God's thoughts and plans are beyond our *human* ability to know. But according to Paul, what do we Christians have in us so that we can see the possibilities God has ahead for us?

_____
_____
_____
_____

Why do you think God wants us to see beyond what is right now to what could be?

_____

_____

_____

_____

_____

It's risky to launch out on a new adventure. What are you most concerned about as you make changes to your lifestyle?

_____

_____

_____

_____

_____

Stephen Arterburn, a Christian counselor and author, points out that life without risk is not much of a life:

> Predictability really can chain us to old things and prevent us from moving toward the new. Comfort can encase us in a womb we should have outgrown but still retreat into. We must give up the chains of predictability and the womb of comfort and jump out there and take a risk if we are to truly live. . . .
>
> We risk connecting, because if we don't, parts of us will die in isolation. We must risk loving again, because if we don't, we will become bitter and isolated. We risk succeeding, knowing it might prove to be a failure and we might look inadequate. If we do not risk, however, we will live horrible lives of boredom and loneliness, convincing ourselves we are okay as we mark time toward a miserable end. It does not have to be that way if we will choose to take a risk.[2]

The possibilities are ahead of us to experience. We just need to remember that God is with us on our journey, and He is always by our side to pick us up when we fall.

Father, I may never be much of a risk-taker, but I'm willing to explore new possibilities, because I have Your promise to be there to catch me when I stumble. I want to move forward in Your capable and loving hands. Amen.

Day
2

PROMISES

Gracious God, every day I am discovering a new promise in the Bible that seems written just for me in my circumstances that day! How wonderfully loving You are and how much I want to cling to those promises and claim them for my own. I thank You for these promises, Lord. Amen.

Read Psalm 18:32-36. What are the nine promises that this particular adventurer (King David) is counting on from God?

1. _____
2. _____
3. _____
4. _____
5. _____
6. _____
7. _____
8. _____
9. _____

One of the most adventurous journeys described in the Bible is the Exodus, when Moses led the Israelites out of Egypt to the Promised Land. What should have been about a two-week journey, though, turned into 40 years of travel. Although God had promised the Israelites that He would lead them to the Promised Land, and though the Israelites had promised to obey God, the people did not always keep their promise. What's worse, they often grumbled and complained along the way. Can you just imagine some of their murmuring?

"What, manna again?"
"My feet hurt!"
"Move again? But we just got here!"
"Are you sure we shouldn't stop and ask for directions?"
"I'm tired of wearing the same old thing!"
"This gives a whole new meaning to 'camping trip'!"
"Are we there yet?"

Perhaps you have heard similar whining on your summer trips. Yet God, despite the fact that He had to endure the ingratitude of His people, and despite the fact that the Israelites often let Him down, always kept His promises. Like the Israelites, we also keep going because God keeps on fulfilling His promises to us along the way. Nancie Carmichael states it this way:

Setting your heart on pilgrimage means keeping your heart set on moving forward. . . .

As the Israelites made their long pilgrimage through the wilderness, they had to get up and walk when God prompted them. They followed His lead and made the journey at His pace. They were guided by the cloud of Jehovah. Whenever the cloud lifted from above the Tabernacle tent, they knew it was time to set out on their journey. Whenever the cloud settled, the Israelites made camp. . . .

While God does not lead us directly—with a visible cloud that lifts and settles as He did the Israelites—He leads us nonetheless. Following His lead means staying the course, setting our hearts on completing the journey, and believing that He is a faithful and trustworthy guide.

Though the journey can be long, one of the great things about being a pilgrim on a pilgrimage is that you're not alone! Yes, God is with us on our pilgrimage, but there are other pilgrims on the path, too. Together, we keep going, no matter what, shoulder to shoulder.[3]

Who are the pilgrims who journey with you as you seek to achieve your First Place 4 Health goals?

_____
_____
_____
_____
_____

How do you help each other keep going?

_____
_____
_____
_____
_____

Great God, I am a pilgrim and I need You to be my guide on the path. Thank You for promising to walk beside me and sometimes even to carry me. Amen.

Day 3

POTHOLES

Loving God, I know that an occasional pothole might appear in my path. Help me survive it without totally collapsing. Help me to remember that no matter where my path may lead, You never leave me to walk it alone. Amen.

It's been said that life can turn on a dime, which means that circumstances can change very quickly or in a very small space. Most often this figure of speech is used to show how life can change its course in an instant. Depending on the situation, that change can be either good or bad—but either way it will be rapid. Have you ever experienced a pothole that caused your path to suddenly twist and turn so that you found yourself on a new path . . . and not one of your choosing?

This type of life-altering pothole is exactly what happened to Naomi and her daughters-in-law Orpah and Ruth when they were all suddenly widowed. Read the first chapter of Ruth. According to verses 8-9, what did Naomi expect Ruth and Orpah to do?

_____

_____

_____

_____

_____

When Orpah and Ruth tried to accompany Naomi, why did Naomi say that they should not come with her (see verses 11-12)?

_____

_____

_____

_____

Orpah eventually decided to stay in Moab, but Ruth took the risk of a new (and possibly dangerous) adventure by accompanying her mother-in-law back to Bethlehem. What did Ruth pledge to Naomi (see verses 16-17)?

_____

_____

_____

_____

David Bordon and Thomas Winters, in their book *God's Road Map for Women,* imagine Ruth and Naomi frozen in that moment of time:

> They stand at the wind-whipped crossroads, their black shawls falling away from their faces to reveal two women wrapped tightly in grief and in each other's embrace. One is young, too young to be mourning the loss of her husband—but that's where her life has led. The face of the other is weathered with age. While a widow never truly gets over the loss of her first love, it's the recent death of her two sons that has broken her heart anew. Now mother-in-law and daughter-in-law face losing each other. Unable to support one another financially, they know they should head separate ways. But their love for each other outweighs both their grief and the fear of the future. Whatever may come, they will face it together. Hands clenched, hearts united, they cling to each other and to the promise that God will meet their needs, no matter how deep the wounds in their hearts or how difficult the road ahead seems to be.[4]

According to verses 20-21, what did Naomi now want to be called, and why did she want to be called that?

At what time of the year did Ruth and Naomi arrive in Bethlehem? (see verse 22)?

Merciful Father, at certain times I have wondered why potholes have changed the course of my life—why things have happened to me and those I love. Help me to learn a powerful lesson from those pilgrims Ruth and Naomi. Amen.

PROVISION

O God, I may not actually be starving, but I sure do feel bereft and needy at times, just like Ruth and Naomi. As You take me to a "new land," also show me Your provision for my needs. Thank You in advance. Amen.

When Naomi and Ruth returned to Bethlehem, they were literally starving. Yet God—the One who had launched them on this new path, after all—had made provision for them to be fed. Read the second chapter of Ruth. What was the practice of gleaning (see verses 2-3)?

_____

_____

_____

_____

_____

Now read Leviticus 19:9-10. What two groups of people does this law benefit? Why are Ruth and Naomi able to benefit from this law?

_____

_____

_____

_____

Who was Boaz, and what was his interest in Ruth (see Ruth 2:1,11-12)?

_____

_____

_____

_____

_____

God not only provided for Naomi and Ruth's physical needs, but He also orchestrated events so that Ruth was able to marry Boaz, a kinsman-redeemer who would then allow her all access to his family and faith. Read Ruth 4:13-14. In what ways did God provide for Ruth? In what ways did God provide for Naomi?

God's provision for Ruth	God's provision for Naomi

Ultimately, God's greatest and most amazing provision was His love, which led Ruth to accompany Naomi on a journey from grief to a new life and love that allowed them to be part of the lineage of Jesus. God has charted your journey with just as much care.

Lord, how completely You want to provide for all who will trust in You.
Thank You for showing me that Your plan includes amazing things ahead!
Be my own kinsman-redeemer and make me part of Your family. Amen.

Day 5

PRESENCE

Father, I know You are with me wherever I go; but sometimes I cannot feel
Your presence, and sometimes I wonder if You would want to be where I
have journeyed. Thank You for never leaving me or forsaking me. Amen.

Embarking on a new adventure is always easier with a traveling companion or, better yet, a guide—someone who has already traveled that path and knows what to expect. This is why God offers His presence to everyone who turns to Him. Do you realize that wherever you currently are—physically, spiritually, emotionally and mentally—you are in the presence of the God who loves you?

Read Psalm 139:7-12. As the psalmist recognizes God's presence, why do you think he lists all kinds of scenarios?

_____

_____

_____

_____

What is the psalmist's conclusion about where he can go from God's Spirit? Can we ever be without the presence of God in our lives?

_____

_____

_____

_____

Author Nancie Carmichael, reflecting on how her own young children often wanted to talk to her privately face-to-face, offers these observations:

> I'm thinking that sometimes God wants to get us one-on-one, just to "talk." In the middle of your own difficulties, maybe your heavenly Father just wants to get you alone, to reassure you that He's there and that everything's going to be all right. Trust Him as a child means coming as you are—with your anger, frustrations, questions, and all. We can enter His presence freely, assured that we're never an interruption. His door is always open to us, no matter what's going on. To trust as a child means we can wait for Him, knowing that in His good time, He will show up.[5]

God is always with us, and we can trust Him to be there for us when we call on Him. Read Isaiah 41:10-13. What commandment does God give three times, and what is the qualifier each time?

Do not _____,   for I am _____

Do not _____,   for I am _____

Do not _____,   I will _____

God is always with us. We can rely on His strength and protection as He takes our hand in His.

God Almighty, I am sometimes full of fear and lacking in faith, but I know that You are with me and that I no longer need to live in fear. From now on, with Your help, I shall go forward in faith. Thank You, Lord. Amen.

Day 6 — REFLECTION AND APPLICATION

Strong Protector, gird me with Your holy armor and help me fight the good fight. I know life can be a battle at times, and though I hate conflict of any kind, I trust in You at my side for protection. Amen.

This week has been all about summoning courage in order to risk new adventures. Think about the last five days and write down a word or phrase that comes to mind as you recall each day's study.

Day 1: Possibilities _____

Day 2: Promises _____

Day 3: Potholes _____

Day 4: Provision _____

Day 5: Presence _____

The courage we need as we look forward to our new adventures comes from God, as does our protection along the way. Author Christin Ditchfield states how John Bunyan described this type of protection:

In the classic allegory, *Pilgrim's Progress,* author John Bunyan describes the journey of a man named Christian from sin and bondage in the City of Destruction to eternal peace and joy in the Celestial City. Along the way, Christian faces many trials that test his faith. At one point, he passes through a dark valley inhabited by hideous demonic beings that hover about, just out of sight. . . . Christian is rescued when a friend comes alongside him and begins quoting the Word of God to him, speaking words of truth and goodness and grace. Words that sing God's praises. The demonic beings are forced to flee, and Christian is set free.[6]

Read Psalm 121:7-8. What are three reminders of God's protection?

1. _____
2. _____
3. _____

How does knowing that God will protect you forever make you feel?

_____
_____
_____
_____
_____
_____

Thank You, Lord, that Your provision and Your protection are not just for a season but are forever. Thank You that even when I stray from You, You never forget me. Amen.

REFLECTION AND APPLICATION

Day 7

Gracious God, I need Your strength because sometimes I feel like giving up or giving in or giving out. I know You know this, and I also know that You will come alongside me and offer me Your strength. I'm counting on it. Amen.

In his song "His Strength Is Perfect," singer and songwriter Steven Curtis Chapman writes that God's strength is perfect when our strength is gone and that He will carry us when we can't carry on.[7] It's pretty normal to get tired when you are traveling. In fact, as you are now halfway through this six-week *Fit and Healthy Summer* study, you may find your-self lagging in discipline, interest or perseverance. But that is exactly why God sent His Spirit: to give us power when we are feeling run down and weary.

Read 1 Corinthians 2:3-5. Even the apostle Paul, who was a brilliant the-ologian and an adventurous missionary, acknowledged a need for power beyond his own. How did Paul feel when he arrived in Corinth (see verse 3)?

_____

_____

_____

_____

As Paul faithfully did what God had called him to do, what happened (see verse 4)?

_____

_____

_____

_____

Why does God choose to empower His people when they get to the end of their own strength (see verse 5)?

_____

_____

_____

_____

As you finish this week, what are some areas of your life where you know that you're weak?

_____

_____

_____

_____

As you conclude this week's study, ask God for His power to invade your life in each of these areas.

> *Dear God, Just as Paul knew that he needed You in order to accomplish anything of value, so I also need You each day just to keep on keeping on. I need Your Holy Spirit, Your power, to invade my life and build me up. Thank You for helping me out on this new adventure toward balanced health and a godly lifestyle. Amen.*

Notes

1. Augustine, quoted in Lucinda Secrest McDowell, *Quilts from Heaven: Parables from the Patchwork of Life* (Nashville, TN: B&H Publishers, 2007), p. 125.
2. Stephen Arterburn, *Healing Is a Choice Devotional: Ten Weeks of Transforming Brokenness into New Life* (Nashville, TN: J. Countryman, 2005), p. 100.
3. Nancie Carmichael, *Surviving One Bad Year: 7 Spiritual Strategies to Lead You to a New Beginning* (Nashville, TN: Howard Books, 2009), p. 125.
4. David Bordon and Thomas J. Winters, *God's Road Map for Women*, (Tulsa, OK: Bordon-Winters, 2006), p. 99.
5. Carmichael, *Surviving One Bad Year,* p. 179.
6. Christin Ditchfield, *A Way with Words: What Women Should Know About the Power They Possess* (Wheaton, IL: Crossway, 2010), pp. 96-97.
7. "His Strength Is Perfect," *sing365.com,* 2000-2007. http://www.sing365.com/music/lyric.nsf/His-Strength-Is-Perfect-lyrics-Steven-Curtis-Chapman/169AA891E2F68E4948256D760014BE4D.

Group Prayer Requests

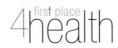

Today's Date: _____

Name	Request

Results

_____

_____

_____

_____

_____

rest stops

Scripture Memory Verse
My soul finds rest in God alone; my salvation comes from him.
Psalm 62:1

When summer is over, are you one of those folks who need a vacation in order to recover from your vacation? Yes, such phrases may be said laughingly, but the sad fact is that many of us use the summer to go, go, go and then wonder why we are so exhausted. Whatever happened to that R & R, or "rest and recreation"? Both are important.

It is definitely advisable to make frequent rest stops on long journeys so you can recharge and refuel for the remaining miles ahead. On our journey toward balanced health and a godly lifestyle, we need to do the same thing. In fact, rest has been proven to be an essential element for restoring physical, mental, emotional and spiritual health. Have you made it part of your summer plans? If not, this week will be a reminder to seek the rest that God alone can give, as our memory verse clearly states.

RETREAT

Day 1

Lord, I want to have a retreat this summer, a time of rest and restoration when I set myself apart and draw close to You. Amen.

Do your summer plans include a retreat? A time and place to intentionally get away from normal responsibilities and distractions and to embrace God's love for you—body, soul and spirit? Read what Pastor Mark Buchanan, in his book *The Rest of God*, says about rest and how it involves a sort of retreat:

In a culture where busyness is a fetish and stillness is laziness, rest is sloth. But without rest, we miss the rest of God: the rest He invites us to enter more fully so that we might know Him more deeply. "Be still, and know that I am God." Some knowing is never pursued, only received. And for that, you need to be still.[1]

It is when you retreat—when you withdraw and are quiet even in the midst of the world's chaos—that you are better able to communicate with God. The concepts of rest, stillness and solitude are ancient spiritual disciplines that were modeled for us by none other than Jesus Christ during His earthly ministry. Read Mark 6:30-32. What were Jesus and His disciples doing?

_____

_____

_____

_____

_____

What did Jesus suggest and guide the disciples to do in the midst of all this activity?

_____

_____

_____

_____

_____

Do you think you don't have time to retreat? Well, if the Savior of the world needed such a rest stop, then who are we to think we can do without? What keeps you from retreating and spending time resting with God?

_____

_____

_____

_____

Sally Breedlove, a speaker and Bible study teacher, writes the following in her book *Choosing Rest: Cultivating a Sunday Heart in a Monday World:*

> We promise ourselves that just around the next corner, life will settle down and we will slow down. But it rarely happens. Why? I believe we are afraid of being alone, afraid of blocks of time when we have nothing we have to do. If rest means entering a space of fearful emptiness, many of us are not sure we want to go there. We may be exhausted, but we'll find something besides rest to fill our fatigue: a video, a nap, a long phone call with a friend. Obviously, these things are not "wrong" but we need to face our own hearts. We are afraid to choose rest because we are afraid of silence, afraid of what we might hear if all sounds were to cease.[2]

What specifically will you do to retreat with God on a regular basis?

_____

_____

_____

_____

Father, I know that only in silence and solitude can I find what You have for me. Help me to retreat to You daily. Amen.

REFUGE

Day **2**

Heavenly Father, help me to remember that when I am distressed, You will shelter and protect me. Thank You for being my refuge. Amen.

This week's memory verse, Psalm 62:1, reminds us that God alone is the One who brings true rest. Write the verse here.

_____

_____

_____

_____

Now read the rest of Psalm 62. After the psalmist states where his own soul finds true rest, he tells God about his worries from enemies who threaten him (see verses 3-4), However, in the midst of his distress, why does he find rest and refuge in God?

_____

_____

_____

_____

What two things does the psalmist admonish people to do (see verse 8)?

1. _____

2. _____

When you hear the word "refuge," what are some similar words that come to mind?

_____

_____

_____

_____

_____

How is the word "refuge" described in these verses?

Psalm 57:1

_____

_____

_____

Psalm 61:3:

_____

_____

_____

Psalm 61:4:

_____

_____

_____

How does the imagery that is used to describe God in Psalm 62 make you feel about drawing close to Him?

_____

_____

_____

_____

_____

Hear my cry, God, when my heart seeks Your shelter and protection from the storms on my journey. Thank You for always hearing me and always responding with Your mighty presence. Amen.

REFRESHMENT

Day 3

O Lord God, how I long to be refreshed, to have my spiritual and physical thirst quenched with the Living Water You have provided for me through Jesus Christ. Help me to rest beside Your quiet waters today so that You may indeed restore my soul. Amen.

One of the reasons that rest stops are important on a long journey is that after a time, travelers are usually in need of refreshment. Read Psalm 23, which describes God as the Shepherd who wants to refresh His flock. According to verses 2-3, how does God refresh us?

_____

_____

_____

_____

_____

In *Traveling Light,* Max Lucado describes the refreshment and the rest that we can find in God:

> The bow cannot always be bent without fear of breaking. For a field to bear fruit, it must occasionally lie fallow. And for you to be healthy, you must rest. Slow down, and God will heal you. He will bring rest to your mind, to your body, and most of all to your soul. He will lead you to green pastures. . . .
>
> And he invites you to rest there. Can you imagine the satisfaction in the heart of a shepherd when, with work completed, he sees his sheep rest in the tender grass?
>
> Can you imagine the satisfaction in the heart of God when we do the same? His pasture is his gift to us. . . .
>
> In a world rocky with human failure, there is a land lush with divine mercy. Your Shepherd invites you there. He wants you to lie down. Nestle deeply until you are hidden, buried, in the tall shoots of his love, and there you will find rest.[3]

What are some refreshing activities you enjoy during the summer?

_____

_____

_____

_____

Fun, family, Frisbees, friends, food and flip-flops can all be ingredients in summer activities, but it's important that our recreation not develop into too much mindless amusement or seeking of entertainment in unhealthy places. Sally Breedlove, in her book *Choosing Rest,* explains the importance of choosing what we do wisely:

> Perhaps we can see the difference between God's true rest and our "rest" by considering the difference between the two words recreation and amusement. Embedded in the root words for

recreation and amusement are vastly different concepts. Recreation is the state of being re-created. It is something we do or choose that fills our soul and body so that we are stronger and richer as a result. Recreation nurtures us. Amusement, on the other hand, literally means "to not think." When we choose amusement we shut down, we disengage. Even more pointed is the ancient meaning of amusement: "to deceive." Could it be that we are deceived when we think that the answer to our weariness is amusement, not recreation? Life is not meant to alternate spasmodically between exhausting, frantic activity and mindless states where we have no energy for anything. We must learn to say no to relentless schedules and cultivate places in our lives for true recreation. Only we can make the choices for what refurbishes our souls and our relationships.[4]

What are some things you can do in order to find rest and refreshment for your soul?

What do you think would happen if you actually refreshed your soul in at least one of these ways?

Lord, I know that sometimes I would rather drown in amusement than seek the true rest that You long to give me. Help me to take a rest stop today and soak up Your goodness and grace. Amen.

Day
4

REPENTANCE

Jesus, lover of my soul, today I ask You to meet me where I am
on this journey and to help me to recognize my need for repentance.
Thank You, Lord, for all that You are doing in my life. Amen.

Imagine that you are taking a road trip from Denver, Colorado, to San
Francisco, California. Obviously, your route would have you driving in
a westward direction. But let's suppose you decide that the road going
east looks ever so much more appealing to you, so you proceed to drive
east toward New York City. Sounds crazy, doesn't it? In fact, someone
could reasonably ask you, "How serious are you really about getting to
San Francisco?"

If you really want to reach that destination, it is imperative that you
turn and head the other way! Could this same question be appropriate
when you appear to be going in the opposite direction from where God
has asked you to go? How serious are you about getting closer to God?
David Bordon and Thomas Winters have this to say about going in the
right direction toward God:

> Everyone makes mistakes and poor choices on occasion. But if
> you're serious about following God, once you recognize you're
> headed the wrong direction, you need to stop, turn around, and
> head the right direction. That's what repentance is. It's more
> than being sorry you've gone the wrong way because you've hurt
> both God and yourself. It's agreeing with God that you need to
> change direction—and then doing it. Whether you consider your
> "detour" big or small is irrelevant. Even a road that leads slightly
> east will never take you west unless it turns back around. Ask
> God today if there's any area of your life that needs a change of
> direction. Then, don't make excuses. Turn around.[5]

Read Isaiah 30:15. In this verse, the prophet Isaiah was chastising the Israelites because they knew what to do—they knew where to find life and

strength—but they kept going their own way. Write down this whole verse, underlining the four "rest stop" gifts that God has for all His people.

_____

_____

_____

_____

Now, think about your own life. What is one practical thing you could do to appropriate each gift into your life?

Repentance

_____

_____

_____

Rest

_____

_____

_____

Quietness

_____

_____

_____

Trust

_____

_____

_____

_I am serious about following You, Lord. I know that my strength
will come through repentance and rest, so today I move forward
in that direction, with Your help. Thank You, Lord. Amen._

RESTORATION

Lord, I have noticed some disturbing symptoms of overload in my life.
Help me to seek the rest and restoration that only You can provide. Amen.

One of the definitions of "restore" is "to put again in possession of something." It is from the Latin word *restaurare*—"to renew, rebuild, alter."[6] On his sabbatical from a busy pastorate, Canadian pastor Mark Buchanan finally faced up to his desperate need for a rest stop from life's chaos:

> The inmost places suffered most. I was losing perspective. Fissures in my character worked themselves here and there into cracks. Some widened into ruptures. I grew easily irritable, paranoid, bitter, self-righteous, gloomy. I was often argumentative: I preferred rightness to intimacy. I avoided and I withdrew. I had a few people I confided in, but few friends.[7]

As he sought the rest of God, Buchanan was so transformed that it both restored him personally and revolutionized his ministry. Are you tired like this? Are you weary? Are you discouraged? Do you wish someone would just order you to go away and sleep for three days?

Read Isaiah 40:28-31. According to this Scripture, where should the weary go for strength?

_____

_____

_____

_____

What are the three results of God's restoration?

1. _____

2. _____

3. _____

In order to be restored, we must actively seek God and place our hope in Him. Unfortunately, there are way too many pilgrims who try to bypass rest stops and eventually burn out on their journey.

Perhaps you have heard the story of one particular wagon train headed west on the Oregon Trail. Because the travelers were Christians, each Sunday the group would observe Sabbath rest and not travel. However, the closer the start of the winter snows came, the more panicked some of them were that if they kept up this practice of resting for a day, they would not reach their destination before the snows began. Others wanted to continue honoring their Sabbath practice. Eventually, the community ended up splitting in two, with one group traveling seven days a week and the other maintaining a day of rest.

So, who arrived in Oregon first? Actually, it was the group who took a day off each week. Both the people and their horses were so rested and restored by their Sabbath observances that they ended up being able to travel much more efficiently the other six days. In *The Rest of God: Restoring Your Soul by Restoring Sabbath,* Mark Buchanan points out an oddity about restoration:

> A curious thing about restoration is that it doesn't need doing. Strictly speaking, life carries on without it. Restoration is an invasion of sorts. . . . Restoration shocks the system. It alters not just our health—it alters our world.[8]

In what ways has restoration altered your world?

_____

_____

_____

_____

_____

Dear God, I will come to You daily for the restoration that only You can give. Help me to soar, even as I rest in You. Amen.

REFLECTION AND APPLICATION

Jesus, I hear You calling me to come to You and be renewed in both my body and my soul. Thank You for the invitation. I may be limping and faltering, but I'm on my way. Amen.

Read Matthew 11:28-30. What invitation did Jesus issue?

_____

_____

_____

_____

If you could respond to Jesus in person, what would you say, and why?

_____

_____

_____

_____

Write down one word that specifies what you most need renewed today in each area of your life.

Mental: _____

Spiritual: _____

Physical: _____

Emotional: _____

Your Lord and Savior still reaches out and invites you to take a much needed rest stop, as Sally Breedlove suggests:

> The voice of Jesus calls for you to begin that journey toward Him, toward rest. Listen as He turns toward you: "Are you tired? Worn out? Burned out on religion? Come to me. Get away with me and you'll recover your life. I'll show you how to take a real rest. Walk with me and work with me—watch how I do it. Learn the un-

forced rhythms of grace. I won't lay anything heavy or ill-fitting on you. Keep company with me and you'll learn to live freely and lightly" [Matthew 11:28-30, *THE MESSAGE*]. Walk with Him, right into your own heart. Watch Him turn all that troubles you into a gateway to rest. Walk with Him. Walk away from the press of oughts and shoulds that crowd your heart and time. Walk with Him—you will find yourself and you will find His rest.[9]

How will you turn away from the press of "oughts" and "shoulds" and just walk with Christ today?

_____

_____

_____

_____

Heavenly Father, too often I give in to the oughts and shoulds,
and I forfeit the ability to live in Your grace and peace. Thank You for
continuing to reach out to me with Your hand of love. Amen.

REFLECTION AND APPLICATION

Day 7

O God, if You—the One who spun the stars into space—can take time for rest,
then certainly I can as well. Help me to know that is a good thing. Amen.

God wants you to enter His true Sabbath rest, a rest described as follows by Peter Scazzero in his book *Emotionally Healthy Spirituality:*

The word *Sabbath* comes from a Hebrew word that means "to cease, to stop working." It refers to doing nothing related to work for a twenty-four hour period each week. Sabbath provides for us now an additional rhythm for an entire reorientation of our lives around the living God. . . . God worked. We are to work. God rested. We are to rest.[10]

Today, your seventh day of study this week, may not actually be your day of rest (Sunday or otherwise). However, do seek to plan a Sabbath in the next few days where you can fully embrace the rest God wants to give you. Read Psalm 62:1,5 and Psalm 91:1. Exactly where does the psalmist find rest, and why?

What is your plan for how you will rest? Describe it briefly below.

Never forget how important rest is. As minister and theology teacher Lynne Baab notes in her book *Sabbath Keeping:*

> During a day of rest, we have the chance to take a deep breath and look at our lives. God is at work every minute of our days, yet we seldom notice. Noticing requires intentional stopping, and the sabbath provides that opportunity. . . . Without time to stop, we cannot notice God's hand in our lives, practice thankfulness, step outside our culture's values or explore our deepest longings. Without time to rest, we will seriously undermine our ability to experience God's unconditional love and acceptance.[11]

Rest, just as God rested.

> *O Lord, I never realized the importance of keeping a Sabbath day every week. Thank You for knowing exactly what I need and making provision for it. Help me to keep a Sabbath and find true rest. Amen.*

Notes

1. Mark Buchanan, *The Rest of God: Restoring Your Soul by Restoring Sabbath* (Nashville, TN: Thomas Nelson Publishers, 2006), p. 3.
2. Sally Breedlove, *Choosing Rest: Cultivating a Sunday Heart in a Monday World* (Colorado Springs, CO: NavPress, 2002), p. 143.
3. Max Lucado, *Traveling Light: Releasing the Burdens You Were Never Intended to Bear* (Nashville, TN: Word Publishing, 2001), p. 45-46.
4. Breedlove, *Choosing Rest*, p. 142.
5. David Bordon and Thomas J. Winters, *God's Road Map for Women* (Tulsa, OK: Bordon-Winters, 2006), p. 176.
6. *Merriam-Webster's Collegiate Dictionary*, 11th ed., s.v. "restore."
7. Buchanan, *The Rest of God*, p. 2.
8. Ibid., p. 150-52.
9. Breedlove, *Choosing Rest*, p. 157.
10. Peter Scazzero, *Emotionally Healthy Spirituality: Unleash a Revolution in Your Life in Christ* (Nashville, TN: Thomas Nelson, 2006), pp. 163-64.
11. Lynne M. Baab, *Sabbath Keeping: Finding Freedom in the Rhythms of Rest* (Downers Grove, IL: InterVarsity Press, 2005), p. 18-19.

Group Prayer Requests

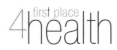

Today's Date: _____

Name	Request

Results

_____

_____

_____

_____

_____

detours

SCRIPTURE MEMORY VERSE

Though I walk in the midst of trouble, you preserve my life; you stretch out your hand against the anger of my foes, with your right hand you save me.

PSALM 138:7

Uh-oh. You started out headed in the right direction. You had a plan. You had a purpose. But first one thing and then another threw you off course, and you had to make a detour. And now you are way off track, wondering if you'll ever find the right road again. Sound familiar?

Let's face it. When we find ourselves on a detour—whether from un-expected troubles, from having made wrong choices or just from having checked out the scenic route—sometimes it takes all we have to follow the detour until we can wind our way back onto the main path. Author and conference speaker Jeanne Zornes put it this way:

> Rocky road is not just a flavor of nutty ice cream. It's the nitty-gritty of life. It's learning that getting where we want isn't always easy. Sometimes life's journey is rutted and rocky and rough. We're not where we want to be, and yet we don't see how things can get any better. God knows all about our despair.[1]

Fortunately, our despair over any of life's detours—those deviations from a direct, expected or previously decided course of action—need not be permanent. Have you strayed from the true path of your faith jour-ney? Have you deviated from the regimen you adopted when you began this *Fit and Healthy Summer* study? Don't despair, for there is truly hope as the psalmist in this week's memory verse points out: God walks with us in the midst of trouble, not only to preserve our lives, but also to reach out a saving hand and pull us back to Him.

Day 1 TROUBLE

Heavenly Father, sometimes it seems as if trouble finds me, even when I'm not looking for it. Please help me listen carefully to You and respond in a way that is obedient and promising. Amen.

How do you know when you're in deep trouble? Read what author Joan Chittister has to say about the troubling detours of life:

> The great interruptions of life leave us completely disoriented. We become lost. The map of life changes overnight and our sense of direction and purpose goes with it. Life comes to a halt, takes on a new and indiscernible shape. Promise fails us and it is the loss of promise that dries in our throats. What was is no more and what is to come, if anything, is unclear.[2]

These sorts of disruptions to our plans—these detours—can be scary. So it's comforting to know that God hears the prayers of those in trouble and saves His people. Read Psalm 107, which was written to celebrate the Israelites' return from their exile in Babylon. It describes four different types of people in trouble and tells how God rescues them: wanderers (verses 4-9), prisoners (verses 10-16), the sick (verses 17-20) and the storm-tossed (verses 23-30). In what kind of trouble did the wanderers find themselves (see verses 4-5)?

_____

_____

_____

_____

_____

What did they do, and how did God respond (see verses 6-7)?

_____

_____

_____

_____

_____

After God saved them, what did the psalmist say the wanderers should do, and why (see verses 8-9)?

_____

_____

_____

_____

_____

Lost, hungry, thirsty and exhausted describe these wanderers—and sometimes that's how we could be described, isn't it? Describe what God's provision is for us when we experience the following troubles:

When we're *lost* (see John 14:6)

_____

_____

_____

_____

When we're *hungry* (see John 6:33,35)

_____

_____

_____

_____

When we're *thirsty* (see John 4:10-14)

_____

_____

_____

_____

_____

When we're *exhausted* (see Matthew 11:28-30)

_____

_____

_____

_____

After one mother went through the harrowing experience of having her daughter accidentally killed by her son, she learned some painful but essential lessons on surviving the detours of life:

> Depression became my friend, in a strange and painful way, a pushy friend I really did not want. But this strange friend made it so clear to me that I couldn't just buck up and feel better, or try harder and do better. I was helpless. My husband could not fix me. My closest friends, who somehow loved me too, could not fix me. And Lord knows I could not fix myself. If I wanted to live in a different place than this dark cloud of fear, anger, and sadness, I had to realize that this burden was way too heavy to carry alone. God and God alone was the One who could take the depression and turn it into something teachable. All I had to do was the hardest thing possible for a person like me: I just had to be willing to give up control and give it to Him, and let Him use this cross in my life. Yes, there was plenty of work I had to do if I wanted to get better. But the first step, before my efforts, was to realize that the essential transformation inside of me would not come through my work, but as a gift of grace from God Himself.[3]

All of us will experience detours at one time or another. As in this mother's case, some of those detours will not be of our own choosing. Yet we can know that no matter what detour we are on or where the path may lead us, we have a God who cares for us and will get us back on course.

O Lord, I have wandered away from the path You set me on so long ago. At times, I have been lost, hungry, thirsty and exhausted. Thank You for always being the One who satisfies. Amen.

TEMPTATION

Day
2

Father, it often seems as if I am tempted on every side and at every turn. Thank You for being the One who understands my struggles and promises to never let me be tempted beyond my ability to overcome. Amen.

Let's face it. There is always another path that looks more tempting. Why ride your bike in the hot sun when you can watch television in an air-conditioned room? Why take time to cut up all that fresh fruit when you can just pull up to the drive-in window and order a big meal? Why awaken early to spend time with God when you can just roll over and sleep a little longer?

One of the biggest detours in life's journey is when we know where God wants us to go but we deliberately choose an alternate path. Thousands of years ago, the Lord spoke to a man named Jonah and asked him to go to a city named Nineveh. Yes, the very Creator of the universe made a verbal request to this man. And still, Jonah chose to make a detour rather than obey.

Read Jonah 1:1-17. What did God ask Jonah to do, and why (see verse 2)?

How did Jonah respond to God (see verse 3)?

_____

_____

_____

_____

What temptation was Jonah giving in to by heading the opposite way?

_____

_____

_____

_____

Can you think of a recent occasion when you were tempted to take the safe or easy way out? If so, what did you do?

_____

_____

_____

_____

As soon as Jonah boarded the ship at Joppa, what consequences occurred (see verses 4-5)?

_____

_____

_____

_____

When confronted, why did Jonah immediately identify himself as a religious man (see verse 9)?

_____

_____

_____

_____

What did Jonah confess, and what did the sailors do (see verses 10-16)?

_____

_____

_____

_____

_____

For someone who was seeking the easy path, how did things get especially complicated (see verse 17)?

_____

_____

_____

_____

_____

God of grace and mercy, help me to own up to my choices and learn from all my mistakes. Thank You that even when I'm in the "belly of a whale," You are using that time to teach me important lessons. Amen.

TURNING

Day
3

Dear Lord, help me to finally get it right after I've first done wrong. May I respond to You in obedience by doing exactly what You say. Thank You for promising to empower me in this way. Amen.

A detour will, by definition, eventually lead us back to where we need to be. It's just an alternate route. Sometimes, though, our choices get us off the straight and narrow, and instead of following along hoping that we'll eventually end up where we need to be, what we need to do is turn completely around. In her book *Hope 4 You*, First Place 4 Health national director Carole Lewis shares such an experience:

When we get lost, it is imperative that we need to get out the map (our Bible), find out where we got off track, and then head back in the right direction. If we have the Word of God deep inside of us, then the Holy Spirit is able to bring it up when we feel hopeless of ever getting back on the right path. . . .

The key is to remember that even when we feel hopelessly lost, God is not lost at all. He knows exactly where He is and where we are, and He has a purpose for everything we go through on the journey. If we have ever walked with Him, we can walk with Him again. The secret is being willing to turn around and go back to the point where we quit walking in step with Him. . . .

Walking with God is, without a doubt, the most exciting journey we could ever undertake. It is never boring or dull, and always full of challenges that demand we stay alert. The most beautiful thing about the journey with Christ is that the longer we walk together, the easier it is to turn around and get back in step.[4]

Read Jonah 2:1-10. What caused Jonah's turnaround, and what did he do (see verses 1-2)?

_____

_____

_____

_____

_____

In verse 3, how did Jonah describe what had happened to him after he chose to disobey God?

_____

_____

_____

_____

_____

What did Jonah conclude from the experience? What did he decide to do as a result (see verse 4)?

_____

_____

_____

_____

What did God do for Jonah when he called out to the Lord (see verses 6-10)?

_____

_____

_____

_____

_____

What are some of your own detour experiences? How has God rescued you from those situations?

_____

_____

_____

_____

_____

Dear Jesus, I will call out to You whenever I have turned from Your way and taken a detour. Sometimes I need Your help to save me from myself! Amen.

TRUTH

Day 4

Father, thank You that detours are not always final if I am open to turning around and starting over again. Thank You for not giving up on me. Amen.

"I'm not going to ask you again!" Have you ever said this to your children or your students? If you have, you probably had expected to be obeyed immediately, and when that didn't happen, you issued this warning, implying that the person would not be given a second chance to obey you. Yet how many times does our heavenly Father give us a second chance to respond properly to His commands?

Read the third chapter of Jonah. Note that the continuation of Jonah's story begins with the words, "Then the word of the LORD came to Jonah a second time." What did God ask of Jonah this time (see verses 1-2)?

_____

_____

_____

_____

What did Jonah do in response to God's command (see verse 3)?

_____

_____

_____

_____

Jonah preached the message God had given him, but no one was more surprised than the messenger at the response of the Ninevites. What did all of the Ninevites do (see verses 5-9)?

_____

_____

_____

What did God do in response (see verse 10)?

_____

_____

_____

_____

Now read the fourth chapter of Jonah. The Ninevites had responded quickly and properly to God's truth, and they received the same mercy and grace that Jonah had been given. However, what was Jonah's response to God's compassionate dealing with the Ninevites (see verses 1-3)?

_____

_____

_____

_____

When was a time you became angry because something you wanted to see happen didn't go your way?

_____

_____

_____

_____

How quickly we forget what God has done for us! Even though we received mercy and grace, it is so easy to become harsh toward others who stand in need of that same mercy and grace. When we are angry or depressed, many of us act like Jonah—we are more concerned about our own comfort than the needs of the people around us. It is only through embracing God's truth that He can and will heal and use us.

Dear heavenly Father, sometimes I forget (or I choose to forget) the truth that Your forgiveness is for everyone, as should my forgiveness be. Help me to obey You and build Your kingdom here on earth. Amen.

TRANSFORMED

Day
5

Change my heart, O God, to make it more and more like You. I relinquish myself to Your care. Please transform me from the inside out. Amen.

Even detours can be redemptive, as they cause us to learn hard lessons and change into stronger, more focused people of God. This radical change from the inside out is godly transformation. Read 1 John 2:10-17. What is the difference between those who walk in darkness and those who live in light?

Walking in darkness	Living in light

In this passage, John is writing to fathers, young men and children to encourage them in holiness. What are the benefits he shares with them?

Your sins _____

You have known _____

You have overcome _____

You are _____

_____ lives in you.

The one who does the will of God will _____.

During this summer, how have the First Place 4 Health practices of Bible study, prayer and Scripture memory contributed to your own spiritual health?

_____

_____

_____

_____

For many of us, we eat to fill an emotional void or to numb ourselves from life's pain. Dr. Linda S. Mintle states the following about this dangerous trend:

Food is easy to abuse because it is cheap, available, tastes good, is physically satisfying, and emotionally comforting. And, unlike true addictions, you can't abstain from the abused substance. Because eating is part of our everyday lives, avoiding it is difficult. In addition, food abuse does not have the stigma attached to it that alcohol and drug abuse has. Perhaps this explains, in part, why eating problems are so prevalent in the church. Christian activities usually involve food. We meet, greet and eat in church. You might say food is the acceptable overindulgence used to numb interpersonal and emotional pain. Food can even become an idol and source of obsession. It can be abused by both those with and without faith.[5]

In what way can food become an idol in our lives? In what ways is it an "acceptable overindulgence"?

God Almighty, I know that You alone can transform me into a strong individual who does not rely on any other person or substance for coping with life's challenges. Thank You, Lord, for Your provision. Amen.

REFLECTION AND APPLICATION

Day 6

I praise You, Lord, because truly You are worthy of all my gratitude for all that You have done and continue to do for me and those I love. Help me to always remember to count my blessings. Amen.

Summer isn't usually the season for making "what I'm thankful for" lists. Yet why should such an exercise only be reserved for November, when we celebrate Thanksgiving Day? Paul wrote to the believers in Ephesus, "I have not stopped giving thanks for you, remembering you in my prayers" (Ephesians 1:16). And he wrote to the church at Philippi, "I thank my God every time I remember you" (Philippians 1:3). What can you thank God for in the middle of an upsetting or perhaps life-altering detour?

_____

_____

_____

_____

When her daughter, Shari, was killed on Thanksgiving Day, Carole Lewis learned an important lesson about the healing power of a thankful heart. As she shares in *Hope 4 You:*

> When we're in the midst of difficult circumstances—shock at the sudden death of a loved one, for example—we often don't realize how a close walk with the Lord prepares us to be thankful. This, to me, is the beauty of memorizing Scripture. Not only have we hidden the truth of God's Word in our heart, but the Holy Spirit also calls it to our attention by bringing a key verse to the surface of our grieving and overwhelmed mind. . . .
>
> At the time of my daughter Shari's death, I never dreamed that thankfulness would be one of the resources God would use to heal the huge void left in my heart. I know that people grieve in different ways and that every one is different, but I have come to believe that being thankful in the midst of tragic circumstances is the key to moving toward healing.[6]

Getting a fresh perspective and realistic worldview may help your attitude on gratitude and enable you to recognize that you are truly blessed if you . . .

- Woke up this morning with more health than illness (up to a billion people around the world are more sick than well).

- Live out the week (millions around the world won't).

- Do not live in danger of battle (people in more than 50 nations have war or conflict at their front door).

- Aren't in prison (millions around the world are incarcerated, with estimates that at least 20 percent are innocent of the charges against them or are being held as political hostages).

- Have enough to eat (20 million people around the world don't).

- Can attend church without fear of harassment, arrest, torture, or death (three billion people in the world cannot).

- Have food in your cupboards or refrigerator, clothes on your back, a roof over your head, and a place to sleep (you are ahead of 75 percent of the world).

- Have money in the bank or your wallet, or even spare change (you are ahead of 92 percent of the world).

- Can read (two billion people around the world cannot).

- Have both parents alive and still married (most people in the United States are not as fortunate).[7]

As you reflect on this week's lessons, what would be your own "thankful list"? List these items below.

_____

_____

_____

_____

_____

_____

Glory to You, O God, for all You are. Thank You for coming alongside me on the journey, and may I always know You as my provider. Amen.

REFLECTION AND APPLICATION

*Heavenly Father, sometimes I get really tired. But I will keep going forward
in faith, for I know that You will help to strengthen and sustain me. Amen.*

Some days all we can do is put one foot in front of the other and travel on.
The lyrics from "Press On," a song performed by Selah, continue to in-
spire many people to do just that: "In Jesus' name, we press on, Dear Lord,
with the prize clear before our eyes, we find the strength to press on."[8]

Today, take some time to refocus your goals on this journey you are
taking toward balanced health. If you have had setbacks during the course
of studying *Fit and Healthy Summer,* now would be a good time to "learn
and turn"—learn valuable lessons and turn back to the path set before you
by God, who not only leads the way but also takes you by the hand.

Read Hebrews 12:1-3. In order to travel on—to keep going forward on
your journey—what must you do?

_____

_____

_____

_____

What entanglements do you need to throw off?

_____

_____

_____

_____

How will fixing your eyes on Jesus help you to keep traveling on and running with perseverance?

_____

_____

_____

_____

What specific plans do you have for getting back on track?

_____

_____

_____

_____

As you conclude this week's study, close your time with the following prayer by Thomas Merton, a well-known author and Trappist monk.

> *God, we have no idea where we are going. We do not see the road ahead of us. We cannot know for certain where it will end. Nor do we really know ourselves, and the fact that we think we are following Your will does not mean that we are actually doing so. But we believe that the desire to please You does in fact please You. And we hope we have that desire in all that we are doing. We hope that we will never do anything apart from that desire. And we know that if we do this You will lead us by the right road, though we may know nothing about it. Therefore, we will trust You always though we may seem to be lost and in the shadow of death. We will not fear, for You are ever with us, and You will never leave us to face our perils alone. Amen.*[9]

Notes

1. Jeanne Zornes, *When I Got on the Highway to Heaven . . . I Didn't Expect Rocky Roads* (Wheaton, IL: Harold Shaw Publishers, 1998), p. 16.
2. Joan Chittister, *Scarred by Struggle, Transformed by Hope* (Grand Rapids, MI: Eerdmans, 2003), p. 1.
3. Mary Beth Chapman, *Learning to See: A Journey of Struggle and Hope* (Grand Rapids, MI: Revell, 2010), p. 69.
4. Carole Lewis, *Hope 4 You: God's Plan for Your Health and Happiness* (Ventura, CA: Regal, 2010), p. 45.
5. Linda S. Mintle, "Body Image and Eating Disorders" in *Praying Through Life's Problems: Inspiring Messages of Hope* (Nashville, TN: Integrity Publishers, 2003), p. 147.
6. Lewis, *Hope 4 You*, p. 97.
7. W.B. Freeman, *The Longer-Lasting Inspirational Bathroom Book* (New York: FaithWords, 2007), p. 57.
8. Dan Burgess, "Press On," *All The Lyrics.com,* 2002-2010. http://www.allthelyrics.com/lyrics/selah/press_on-lyrics-219211.html (accessed October 7, 2010).
9. Thomas Merton, *Thoughts in Solitude* (New York: Noonday Press, 1987), p. 83.

Group Prayer Requests

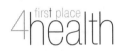

Today's Date: _____

Name	Request

Results

_____

_____

_____

_____

_____

_____

destination

SCRIPTURE MEMORY VERSE
I am still confident of this: I will see the goodness of the LORD in the land of the living.
PSALM 27:13

"This world is not my home, I'm just passing through."[1] So say the words to an old gospel hymn, and so says God Himself. The true destination of every Christ follower is heaven, where all who believe will enjoy God's gift of eternal life.

However, even though this earthly realm is not our final destination, it is the place that we inhabit for this segment of our journey. And God's provision for each of us includes, not only the hope of heaven, but also His goodness "in the land of the living," as this week's memory verse says.

Our responsibility becomes, then, not only securing assurance that because we have placed our faith in Christ Jesus, we will spend eternity with Him (John 3:16), but also choosing to walk with Christ each day—living fully in His grace and mercy. And making intentional decisions for balanced health—spiritual, physical, emotional and mental—is both an act of obedience and a gift from God.

HOPE
Day 1

Gracious God, I want to cling to You as I move forward toward my ultimate destination. Thank You for the hope You bring into every situation. Amen.

According to Carole Lewis, "You and I have DNA that is hardwired for hope. . . . No other living, breathing, creature, except humans, was created to have hope. . . . None of us can survive long without hope."[2]

Read Psalm 33:20-22. What two words are used to describe the Lord?

Our _____

Our _____

Which of these aspects of God's character do you need the most today, and why?

_____

_____

_____

_____

_____

What four action words (verbs) are used to describe our lives as people of hope?

1. _____
2. _____
3. _____
4. _____

What does the psalmist know about God's love that allows him to hold on to hope?

_____

_____

_____

_____

_____

Chesed is the Old Testament Hebrew word that is translated in this passage as "unfailing love" (it is also sometimes translated "lovingkindness"). Yet even those words cannot encompass the actual greatness of

God's love. How does allowing God's unfailing love to rest on you give you hope?

_____

_____

_____

_____

O Lord, thank You for loving me with the greatness of Your unfailing love.
I know I don't deserve it, but I accept it as a gift from You today. Amen.

HOLY

Day
2

Most holy God, You know that I don't always feel very holy,
but I do want to be someone who is set apart for Your use. Please
fill me with all I need to serve and speak for You. Amen.

Being holy is not a popular concept in this day and age, probably due to the fact that for many, "holiness" has a connotation of a "holier-than-thou" attitude or someone who lords over others with their personal piety. This connotation, however, could not be further from the truth! To be holy means to be set apart for a special use. In her book *Set Apart,* author and speaker Jennifer Kennedy Dean writes:

> Throughout the Old Testament . . . God conferred holiness upon something, then worked that holiness out in practice. To be holy meant to be set apart for God's use—whether person, animal, day, or instrument. . . .
>
> God brings that same definition of holiness right into the New Testament and makes it the centerpiece of the new kingdom. You are holy because God has declared you so, has cleansed you with the eternal blood of the Lamb, and is now working out that holiness.[3]

Read 1 Peter 1:14-16. Most of us interpret these words as a command. However, if you read them as a promise, how do they make you feel?

_____

_____

_____

_____

Now turn to Micah 6:8. What three holy acts does the Lord require of His people?

1. _____

2. _____

3. _____

Think of your own life and circumstances today. In the space below, fill in one specific way you could act on each command.

Act justly

_____

_____

_____

_____

Love mercy

_____

_____

_____

Walk humbly with God

_____

_____

_____

_____

Father, thank You that You empower me to act justly, love mercy and walk humbly with You as I grow more and more in godliness and faith. Amen.

HEALED

Jehovah Rapha, truly You are the God that heals me—and I'm counting on it! May I willingly participate with You in the process and may I move forward today with new strength. Amen.

Have you ever fallen prey to secret eating—perhaps wolfing down some junk food for a "quick fix"? This usually happens as a reaction to some sort of rejection or painful experience. Some of us who struggle with emotional eating do so by seeking comfort in food in order to fill a void or need that only God can fill.

On our journey with God toward balanced health, many of us have discovered that one reason we have struggled is that we also turn to things other than God to fill a need. What we really need is emotional healing. And God is the very One who can do that! He is known as "Jehovah Rapha"—the God who heals. Healing of this sort requires us to end certain behaviors and initiate new ones. But the first step is to turn to the great healer.

Read Psalm 30:1-2. What two things did the psalmist, the afflicted person, do?

1. _____
2. _____

What are three specific things God has done for him?

1. _____
2. _____
3. _____

In his book *Journey into Healthy Living*, Scott Reall, founder of Restore Ministries for the YMCA, says this about healing and recovery:

> First, we must make peace with God, peace with ourselves, and peace with others. . . . When we're at peace, we can grow into new creatures with new approaches to living. God transforms us from the inside out, producing new relationships with food and our bodies. Old, destructive patterns change, and we become different; we have different friends, different lifestyles, different goals. . . .
>
> Recovery should involve many new things—new friends, new environments, and new food choices. This won't happen overnight; it's a process that will take time. . . . You're not striving for perfection—you want progress. You might take two steps forward, and then one step back. You will have setbacks and slips, times when you fall back into a previous pattern. There's a difference between a brief slip and a major, full-blown relapse. . . .
>
> Build your program for change around God and the people supporting you. Know that you can change with God's help and the help of others. Say good-bye to old habits and replace them with new, healthier ones.[4]

What are a few areas in your life where you know you need God's healing?

_____

_____

_____

_____

_____

What are a few habits that you need to change?

_____

_____

_____

_____

What new habits can you begin to replace these?

_____
_____
_____
_____

*Jesus, I know this journey is a process sometimes of three steps forward
and two steps back, but at least I'm moving forward with Your help.
Thank You for giving me signs of progress along the way. Amen.*

HIS

Day 4

*Sometimes I wonder, God, who I am. There are so many different opinions
about me from so many people. Help me to hear only Your voice. Amen.*

One reason so many people struggle with insecurity and low self-esteem is that they find their identity only through what others think of them or what the culture says about them. Friends, that is a fast track to self-destruction! Our goal is to get to a healthy place where we are defined by our relationship to our Creator and thus known as a child of God, beloved, or chosen one.

Read Romans 8:14-18 and complete the following:

People who are led by God's Spirit are . . .

_____
_____
_____

If we live in fear, then we act like . . .

_____
_____
_____

If we live by the Spirit, we act like . . .

_____

_____

_____

According to verse 16, how do we know we are God's children?

_____

_____

_____

_____

According to verse 17, those who belong to God are His "heirs." What two things do we inherit from God?

1. _____

2. _____

The apostle Paul, who wrote this letter to the church at Rome, knew both experiences. What does he say about these inheritances (see verse 18)?

_____

_____

_____

_____

We are God's beloved. We belong to Him—we are His—and He loves us. So don't fall into the trap of believing lies from those who would tell you otherwise. Scott Reall shares the following about his growth in this area:

> You can't love part of yourself and not another; it's inner dis-cord. So if the enemy can accomplish that by making you hate your body, his work is halfway done, his first lie accepted. But God wants you to know the truth. He is saying, "I made you—all of you. Everything about you. And I love you." The journey to

loving everything about yourself—your flaws and your gifts—is foundational. In my own personal journey of recovery, I needed to believe the truth that God loves me with all the mistakes that I've made, with all of my flaws. My relationship with God is central in my life, because I know He loves me unconditionally. The standard that I judge myself by is no longer coming from the world, but from God who created me.[5]

It is easy to get overly critical of ourselves—especially when we feel that we are not progressing in the journey the way that we think we should—but we need to always remember that we belong to God and that He loves us for who we are.

> *Thank You, Lord, for delivering me from a spirit of fear into a spirit of Sonship! I know beyond the shadow of a doubt that You love me unconditionally, and I accept Your love into my whole being. Amen.*

HUNGER

Day 5

> *May I be hungry for more of You, Lord, and not for those things which only satisfy in a temporary way. Today I ask that You give me discernment and strength to pursue the right path. Amen.*

The First Place 4 Health program provides many aids—nutrition guidelines, menu plans and the Live It Trackers, to name just a few—to help you develop good eating habits. You know to avoid empty calories and quick fixes. But what about your hunger for that which is not food?

Read Matthew 5:6. As part of His Sermon on the Mount, what did Jesus promise to all who hunger?

What does hungering for righteousness look like?

_____

_____

_____

_____

Jen Hatmaker, a young mother, came to this conclusion about hunger:

> As a whole, mankind is driven by hunger. . . .
>
> You will be filled by whatever you're hungry for. Contentment is not a matter of God being capable of satisfying us. His end of the deal is 100 percent guaranteed. He told us literally hundreds of times in Scripture that those who hunger for Him will be satisfied. Period. It's a nonnegotiable. . . .
>
> If you don't have godly contentment, you aren't hungry for it. You are starved for something else, and it has left you spiritually malnourished. . . .
>
> What are you starved for? Money? Attention? Power? Validation? Status?
>
> My appetite has wandered to the same junk food for years: approval. . . . It has certainly distracted me from enjoying satisfaction in God because I was too busy trying to find it in the opinions of others.
>
> I don't know what you hunger for. . . . There is one, and only one, source for complete contentment, and that's God. We need to _develop a hunger_ for Him. That's our part. Let's let Him worry about satisfying it.[6]

Other than food, what do you hunger for, and why?

_____

_____

_____

_____

What strategies have you developed to satisfy your hunger for righteousness?

_____

_____

_____

_____

_____

_____

> *Father God, I renounce the tendency that I have to seek approval from everyone else in my life except You. Deep down, You know that I want to please You and live a holy life. Thank You, Lord, for helping me pursue the path of righteousness. Amen.*

REFLECTION AND APPLICATION

Day 6

Gracious and loving God, I need to know Your comfort and Your safety. I ask You to stay with me and hold me in Your love. Thank You, Lord, that You are always with us. Amen.

Robert Munsch wrote a poignant picture book for children of all ages called *Love You Forever.* The book begins with a mother holding her newborn son while singing, "I'll love you forever, I'll like you for always, as long as I'm living my baby you'll be."

The story progresses, with the little boy growing up into a man; and throughout each stage of life, the mother holds the son and repeats those words. At the end, however, when the mother is old and sick, the son holds his small mother, rocking her in his arms and singing to her, "I'll love you forever, I'll like you for always, as long as I'm living my Mommy you'll be."[7] Life has come full circle, and the one who was held is now doing the holding.

Being held by someone who is telling you how much you are loved is both the most comforting and most secure feeling of all.

Read Psalm 73:23-24. As the psalmist journeys through life, what four truths does he cling to along the way?

1. _____
2. _____
3. _____
4. _____

Which of these truths brings you the most comfort, and why?

_____
_____
_____
_____

For a little musical comfort, go to the Internet and find a version of Natalie Grant singing the song "Held." In the song, she states, "This is what it means to be held . . . to know that the promise was that when everything fell we'd be held."[8] What was a time during this summer when "everything fell" and God held you?

_____
_____
_____
_____

*Dear God, hold me in Your arms today. Thank You for knowing what
I need next and for showing me the right way to go. Amen.*

Day 7

REFLECTION AND APPLICATION

*Father in heaven, I look forward to one day seeing You face to face. Meanwhile,
help me walk the road here on earth with dignity and obedience. Amen.*

Congratulations! You have reached at least one destination this summer: completing *Fit and Healthy Summer*! In the space below, reflect on what significant lessons have been revealed to you and the accomplishments you have made in each of the four keys areas of healthy living:

Physical

_____
_____
_____
_____

Spiritual

_____
_____
_____
_____

Mental

_____
_____
_____
_____

Emotional

_____
_____
_____
_____

The book of Revelation does just that: it *reveals*. Through vibrant imagery, it presents a picture of our real home—the final destination for all Christ-followers. Read Revelation 22:3-5. What things will we see in heaven?

_____
_____
_____
_____

What will there *not* be in heaven?

_____

_____

_____

_____

What part of this picture gives you the greatest anticipation?

_____

_____

_____

_____

The most important thing about our being in heaven will be, of course, the fact that our long journey will be over. We will finally be home with God. Max Lucado describes what will happen:

> By that moment only one small bag will remain. Not guilt. It was dropped at Calvary. Not the fear of death. It was left at the grave. The only lingering luggage will be this God-given longing for home. And when you see him, you'll set it down. Just as a returning soldier drops his duffel when he sees his wife, you'll drop your longing when you see your Father. Those you love will shout. Those you know will applaud. But all the noise will cease when he cups your chin and says, "Welcome home." And with scarred hand he'll wipe every tear from your eye. And you will dwell in the house of your Lord—forever.[9]

Until that day comes, keep on course and persevere in your quest to lead a healthy and balanced life for the Lord!

> *Dear Lord, please bless me and keep me. Shine Your face upon me*
> *and be gracious to me. Turn Your face toward me and give me peace*
> *(see Numbers 6:24-26). Amen.*

Notes

1. Albert E. Brumley, "This World Is Not My Home," *LetsSingIt®*, 1997-2010. http://artists.letssingit.com/charlie-walker-lyrics-this-world-is-not-my-home-c2gzr6r.

2. Carole Lewis, *Hope 4 You: God's Plan for Your Health and Happiness* (Ventura, CA: Regal, 2010), p. 9.

3. Jennifer Kennedy Dean, *Set Apart: A 6-Week Study of the Beatitudes* (Birmingham, AL: New Hope Publishers, 2009), p. 13.

4. Scott Reall, *Journey into Healthy Living: Freedom from Body Image and Food Issues* (Nashville, TN: Thomas Nelson, 2008), p. 53.

5. Ibid., p. 33-34.

6. Jen Hatmaker, *Road Trip: Five Adventures You're Meant to Live* (Colorado Springs, CO: NavPress, 2006), p. 136.

7. Robert Munsch, *Love You Forever* (Buffalo, NY: Firefly Books Ltd., 1995), p. 2,26.

8. Christa Wells, "Held," *eLyrics.net*, 2000-2010. http://www.elyrics.net/read/n/natalie-grant-lyrics/held-lyrics.html.

9. Max Lucado, *Traveling Light: Releasing the Burdens You Were Never Intended to Bear* (Nashville, TN: Word Publishing, 2001), p. 159.

Group Prayer Requests

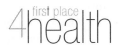

Today's Date: _____

Name	Request

Results

_____

_____

_____

_____

_____

_____

Fit & Healthy Summer
leader discussion guide

Fit and Healthy Summer is a six-week long Bible study, with one group meeting per week, and is recommended for any member who has completed at least one regular First Place 4 Health session. This shorter study has been specifically designed for First Place 4 Health members who desire to maintain healthy habits during the summer months, when breaks in normal routines can prove challenging to maintaining normal fitness and health routines. It can also be done individually as a personal study by anyone on a journey to balanced health.

For in-depth information, guidance and helpful tips about leading a successful First Place 4 Health group, spend time studying the *First Place 4 Health Leader's Guide*. In it, you will find valuable answers to most of your questions, as well as personal insights from many First Place 4 Health group leaders.

For the group meetings in this session, be sure to read and consider each week's discussion topics several days before the meeting—some questions and activities require supplies and/or planning to complete. Also, if you are leading a large group, plan to break into smaller groups for discussion and then come together as a large group to share your answers and responses. Make sure to appoint a capable leader for each small group so that discussions stay focused and on track (and be sure each group records their answers!).

Following are some discussion questions for each of the six group meetings.

week one: maps

During this first week, welcome the members to your group and collect the Member Surveys. Begin your Bible study time with a prayer, asking God to illuminate the heart and mind of each participant.

Discuss what is usually the hardest task you have to do when preparing for a summer trip. What about as you begin this study?

Spend some time sharing how discipline regarding exercise is either working for you or not (see Day 3). Have the group share some ideas and encouragement for a summer strategy in this area.

Discuss how during the next six weeks, the group will be seeking ways to pursue balanced health. Share what you wrote for "My part" and "God's part" on Day 5.

Talk about who are your "enemies" on this journey (see Day 6). Who or what might try to prevent the members from reaching their goals for a fit and healthy summer?

Ask the members if it was difficult to think of what God might say to them (see Day 7). How could they better understand God's unconditional love and delight in them, His children? Go around and have some in the group share their favorite God-loves-me verses from the Bible.

week two: baggage

Ask who in the group is the kind of person who can always get by with only carry-on luggage? Who in the group is the type who has to sit on your suitcase to make it close? What color is their luggage? Why did they choose it?

Just as King David gave in to the desires of his flesh, so do we on numerous occasions (see Day 1). Share a time when that has happened to you, and what the consequences were.

According to Max Lucado, God says of our extra baggage, "I'll carry that one." Lucado also encourages us to get rid of guilt and other sinful baggage that is weighing us down and holding us back (see Day 3). Discuss why this is often so hard to do?

Discuss how accepting God's forgiveness and forgiving ourselves can bring us true freedom (see Days 4 and 5). Ask the members if there are any ways they are still acting like those freed slaves in Texas who were ignorant of the Emancipation Proclamation.

Ask the members what kind of encouragement and fellowship they most need when they are burdened on life's journey (see Day 6). What tangible ideas can your group try with one another during this session to fulfill that need?

week three: new adventures

Ask the members if they have ever taken a trip that was risky or dangerous (see Day 1). If so, have them describe the situation. How did they grow from that experience?

Discuss what promises of God the members are counting on during this *Fit and Healthy Summer* journey (see Day 2). What Scripture verses share those promises?

Share a time when you encountered a "pothole" that changed your life path so much that you ended up down a route that you never would have chosen (see Day 3). How did God provide in that situation?

Ask members to recall a time when God seemed absent or at least very far away (see Day 5). Why do they think that happened? What do they believe now about God's presence on their journey?

Discuss how this summer's quest for balanced health and a godly lifestyle is different from other ventures where they might have relied on willpower alone (see Day 7). Ask the members who they know who has accomplished the "impossible" through the power of God in him or her. (Their answers may include personal or biblical examples, such as the apostle Paul in the Day 7 study.)

week four: rest stops

Go around your group and share specific plans each person has to get some rest and recreation during this summer.

Share your biggest hindrances to incorporating rest, refuge and refreshment into your life (see Days 1–3). As you share the problem, identify whether the solution is or is not within your control.

On Day 3, the group examined Psalm 23, which describes how God helps us to find rest and refreshment for our souls. Have the members choose one thing and share what would happen if they actually did it. (For example, they may have decided to look at their life's activities, and when they did, they realized that they were way too overcommitted. So, they have now decided to cut back on some things when the school season begins this fall.)

Discuss any ways the members have been "driving east" when God called them to "go west" (see Day 4). What area in their lives calls for a change of direction? What are they going to do about it?

Talk about whether the fact that we are to rest just as God rested brings the members great relief or great anxiety. What will it take for them to intentionally stop and experience God's unconditional love and acceptance? Share your hopes and plans for making rest part of your life this week.

week five: detours

Have the group share a time when they wandered off God's prescribed path for their lives (see Day 2)? What specific temptations caused that detour, and what were the results?

Ask the participants if there are any areas of their lives that call for a 180 degree turnaround (see Day 3). How did Carole Lewis's words, "If we have ever walked with Him, we can walk with Him again," encourage them? Where can they begin?

On Day 4 we read that Jonah begged God, "It is better for me to die than to live" (Jonah 4:3) Discuss how when we get depressed or angry, the truth of God's grace and mercy can deliver us from that potentially dangerous detour.

Share how John Newton, a former slave trader, wrote in his hymn "Amazing Grace," "Through many dangers, toils and snares, I have already come." Ask the group to consider some of the trials through which they have come and share one item from their "thankful list" in Day 6.

Discuss what are some tried-and-true methods for getting back on track and continuing forward toward balanced health—physically, mentally, spiritually, and emotionally (see Day 7). Have each person share one or two practical ideas.

week six: destination

This week's memory verse speaks of having confidence. Ask the members what helps them to be confident and hopeful people. What prevents them from always being this way?

Ask the group if they have ever turned to something else to fill a need that only God can fill. What did the Day 3 lesson say would help with healing their emotions?

Ask the members to share if they feel that they live as a beloved child of God or more like an orphan—someone who has no heavenly Father (see Day 4)? Why?

In the Day 5 study, one woman wrote how she hungered for the junk food of approval. Ask the members if they have ever defined themselves by the opinions of others. Why is that a dangerous path?

Conclude by discussing the member's thoughts about heaven (see Day 7). When they think of heaven—the eternal home for all Christ-followers— what images, feelings, promises and longings come to mind (Day 7)? How can they be sure of their final destination?

summertime
helps

Summer can be a challenging time in terms of sticking to your goals to lead a healthier and more balanced lifestyle. Schedules change and routines are broken, and these disruptions can lead to a break in your commitments if you are not adaptable to change. Below are some helpful hints for how you can make good nutrition a stable part of your routine and keep on track during the summer months.

Follow These Summer Eating Tips

- **Be meat savvy.** Choose lean cuts of beef, including round, sirloin and loin cuts. Tenderize the meat to increase flavor and texture without adding fat. Marinate in salsa, low-calorie salad dressing, wine or citrus juices.

- **Seek alternatives.** Items such as gilled chicken breasts, turkey tenders and lamb kabobs make great alternatives to high-sodium hot dogs and hamburgers.

- **Aim for variety.** Kick up the health factor of grilling by adding vegetables and fruits to the menu. Make kabobs with fruit and grill on low heat until the fruit is hot and slightly golden. These healthy snacks will make consuming the recommended daily fruit and vegetable intake much simpler.

- **Stay hydrated.** Summer heat can cause dehydration, so drinks lots of water when the temperatures soar. Add slices of lemons or strawberries to add some natural flavor, or make a batch of *Basil Lemonade* (see recipe on page 156).

- **Keep it simple.** Focus on snacks that don't take a lot of prep work. Keep fresh berries in the refrigerator to add to salads, yogurt and ice creams. Wash fresh green beans and dip in yogurt or low-fat cottage cheese. Keep healthy extras, such as lettuce and tomatoes, in your produce bin. Cut up raw vegetables to serve with low-fat dips. Also try making homemade popsicles by freezing 100 percent juice.

- **Be smooth.** Fruit smoothies are a snap to make. Just toss some fresh fruit, yogurt and milk in your blender.

Have a Very Berry Summer

- **Salads.** Summer is an ideal time for having fresh berries available in the supermarket or at local produce stands. Add berries to mixed greens to make a tasty salad or mix them with other fruits.

- **Parfaits.** Enjoy berries just as they are with all of their summer goodness or layer them with vanilla yogurt and granola to make a parfait.

- **Save for later.** Store blueberries in the freezer to use throughout the winter months. After washing the berries, lay them on top of paper towels to dry and then transfer to a cookie sheet with sides. Place the berries in the freezer for one to two hours and then remove and put in freezer bags or containers. By freezing them in this way, they will break apart more easily.

Try These Light Summer Treats

- **Fudgesicles:** Cool off guilt-free with a fudgesicle—one serving has no fat and just 65 calories.

- **Fruit salsa:** Make a fruit salsa by using whatever fruits you have on hand—such as mangoes, honeydew and cantaloupe—and adding cilantro, chopped onions and a squeeze of lime to taste. Use the salsa on grilled fish instead of butter, as a fat-free salad dressing, or eat it with chips.

- **Veggie kebabs:** Almost any vegetable or fruit can be grilled—zucchini, bell peppers, corn and even spinach. Cooking will bring out the flavor of the vegetable.

- **Watermelon:** People assume that because watermelon is sweet, it must have a lot of sugar. However, two cups of watermelon contain just 92 calories. Try serving the fruit in a salad with mint, onions and feta, or sprinkle salt or chili on fresh-cut watermelon to bring out its natural sweetness.

- **Shrimp cocktail:** Four large shrimp are just 22 calories and contain five grams of protein. A dab of cocktail sauce adds only 30 calories.

- **Iced green tea:** Skip the latte and have an iced green tea. Toss frozen berries or slices of nectarine into your glass—they act as a natural sweetener.

FUN AND HEALTHY
SUMMER ACTIVITIES

Lazy, hazy, crazy days of summer! Let's hope only for the hazy and crazy and not the lazy. Summer can actually be a time to take your family fitness commitments to the next level, as the season actually lends itself to that sense of adventure! Summer is a perfect time to get out of the typical routine and involve your family in creative indoor and outdoor activities. Try some of these for happy, healthy family time.

Do Some Creative Walking

Researchers tell us that 50 percent of men and women who want to stay healthy choose walking as their form of exercise. Regardless of your fitness level or the season of the year, walking is still a great place to start in building a fitness routine. What makes walking so great is that it is inexpensive, it can be done anywhere, and it doesn't require practice or special equipment. Even during the sizzling summer months, walking can be done safely with proper hydration. The following are some creative walking ideas that you might want to build in to your personal summer fitness routine.

- **Take your camera for a walk.** We all live in unique neighborhoods, so as you are taking your daily walk, bring your camera along and take pictures of some of your favorite things about your neighborhood. Record what catches your eye. It could be a beautiful view, a blossoming tree, new neighbors, or a dog taking his owner for a walk. Of course, asking permission to snap a picture is always a good idea. Observe things out of the ordinary. Your walk will go by in no time!

- **Do some neighborhood clean-up.** When you go out walking, take your children or grandchildren along in addition to a small garbage bag. As you walk, pick up the trash in the gutters and along the road. (Wear gloves when you do this.) This is a great way to meet people in your neighborhood and clean up the roads at the same time. Most people are appreciative of someone on a neighborhood clean-up campaign, and they may want to join in.

- **Dribble a basketball.** Dribbling a basketball is a great cardiovascular exercise that will greatly strengthen and improve your hand-and-eye coordination. Take a basketball along on your walk and try to dribble it the whole time. You will be amazed at how hard it is, as it requires a lot of concentration. Of course, be sure to pay attention to where you are walking as you do this!

Go on a Summer Expedition

Take your children on a special summer expedition, such as out to pick berries or apples. All of the walking, stooping, stretching, reaching and bending will provide you with great exercise, and it will also serve as a great learning experience for your children, who will get to see how fresh fruit is grown and harvested. Later, you can enjoy the fruits of your labor with this simple fresh berry recipe:

Baked Berry Dessert
4 cups fresh berries
2 tsp. light margarine
5 macaroon cookies, crushed fine (the hard, crunchy kind)

Wash the berries well and place them in a glass 2-quart baking dish. Slice the margarine into thin pieces and place it on top of the fruit. Sprinkle crumbs over top. Bake at 350° F for 30 to 45 minutes and serve warm. This dessert has only 137 calories and 4 grams of fat.

Take in the Sights

Take advantage of the good summer weather and get some exercise by taking a leisurely stroll along a nature trail or along a scenic road. You can also visit a park with a walking trail and take a few laps to reap some cardiovascular benefits.

Have a Car Wash

Remember the days before the automated car wash? Relive those times by setting aside one day a week for you and your children to wash your car. Working hard together is a great family exercise and all of the scrubbing, reaching and washing provide a great upper body workout. If you are feeling ambitious, ask family and friends if you can wash their cars during summer events while they are visiting. This will serve as a great way to teach your children about important acts of service, and it can also be a part of your "clean up the neighborhood" campaign. For added fun, when you are finished washing the car, turn the hose on the kids!

Take a Bike Ride

Biking is the perfect outdoor activity for nice weather, and you don't even need to own any equipment to enjoy it. Many local bike shops rent bikes and safety gear, and they will even fit you with a helmet and pads to ensure you are wearing them correctly.

Go Bowling

Don't forget the local bowling alley if you live in one of those places where not every day during the summer is a sunny one (you poor folks in Seattle come to mind). Bowling is a great activity to do on a rainy day and will provide you with some exercise. Throw on the goofy shoes and partake in a little competition with your kids.

Have Some Pool Time

If you live in a complex with a pool, you need look no further for some great summer exercise. Most communities also have local pools that will be open for you and your kids to enjoy. Try to avoid going to the pool during mid-day when the sun is the hottest, and be sure to use plenty of sunscreen to protect your skin.

Fast from the Media

Studies show that children are now spending between 28 and 38 hours each week either watching television or being on the computer. While both of these can be educationally beneficial, studies also show that this much sedentary time can contribute to obesity in children and adults. So this summer, challenge your family (and yourself) to go without television or video games for one week a month.

You will be amazed at all the active and creative ways you find to spend time together. This media fast will provide you with opportunities for exercise and family conversation as well as reading and game time. You will also find that your productivity will increase and you will be able to get to all those projects you wanted to do over the summer!

Read a Story from the Bible

As you are doing all of these fun summer activities to keep your physical body in shape, make sure to keep your and your kids' spiritual self in shape as well. If you are not already doing so, take advantage of the fact that your kids are out of school by taking a few minutes at bedtime to read a story from the Bible to them. Make it fun and interesting by paraphrasing the story in your own words or reading from a Bible storybook. Also be sure to spend some time in the Word each day yourself and not let the busyness of summer alter this important priority.

First Place 4 Health
summer menus & recipes

Each menu plan is based on approximately 1,400 to 1,500 calories per day. All recipe and menu exchanges were determined using the Master-Cook software, a program that accesses a database containing more than 6,000 food items prepared using the United States Department of Agriculture (USDA) publications and information from food manufacturers. As with any nutritional program, MasterCook calculates the nutritional values of the recipes based on ingredients. Nutrition may vary due to how the food is prepared, where the food comes from, soil content, season, ripeness, processing and method of preparation. For these reasons, please use the recipes and menu plans as approximate guides. Consult a physician and/or a registered dietitian before starting a weight-loss program.

For those who need more calories, add the following to the 1,400-calorie plan:

- 1,800 calories: 2 ounce equivalent of meat, 3 ounce equivalent of bread, ½ cup vegetable serving, 1 tsp. fat

- 2,000 calories: 2 ounce equivalent of meat, 4 ounce equivalent of bread, ½ cup vegetable serving, 3 tsp. fat

- 2,200 calories: 2 ounce equivalent of meat, 5 ounce equivalent of bread, ½ cup vegetable serving, ½ cup fruit serving, 5 tsp. fat

- 2,400 calories: 2 ounce equivalent of meat, 6 ounce equivalent of bread, 1 cup vegetable serving, ½ cup fruit serving, 6 tsp. fat

First Week Grocery List

Produce
- [ ] arugula
- [ ] banana
- [ ] basil, fresh
- [ ] blueberries
- [ ] carrots
- [ ] celery
- [ ] cherry tomatoes
- [ ] chives, fresh
- [ ] cilantro, fresh
- [ ] eggplant
- [ ] garlic, fresh
- [ ] ginger, fresh
- [ ] grape tomatoes
- [ ] green beans
- [ ] green cabbage
- [ ] green chilies
- [ ] green grapes, seedless
- [ ] green onions
- [ ] green salad
- [ ] green tomato
- [ ] lemons
- [ ] limes
- [ ] mushrooms
- [ ] onion
- [ ] oranges
- [ ] oregano, fresh
- [ ] parsley (flat leaf), fresh
- [ ] plum tomato
- [ ] red onion
- [ ] red pepper
- [ ] romaine lettuce
- [ ] rosemary, fresh
- [ ] shallots
- [ ] tarragon, fresh
- [ ] thyme, fresh
- [ ] tomatoes
- [ ] wax beans, fresh
- [ ] zucchini

Baking Products
- [ ] baking powder
- [ ] baking soda
- [ ] brown sugar
- [ ] canola oil
- [ ] flour, all-purpose
- [ ] flour, whole-wheat
- [ ] nonstick cooking spray
- [ ] olive oil, extra-virgin
- [ ] powdered sugar
- [ ] phyllo dough
- [ ] salt
- [ ] sugar
- [ ] toasted sesame oil
- [ ] vanilla extract

Spices
- [ ] black pepper
- [ ] Cajun seasoning, salt-free
- [ ] chili powder
- [ ] cinnamon
- [ ] cumin
- [ ] garlic powder
- [ ] nutmeg
- [ ] paprika
- [ ] thyme, dried

Nuts/Seeds
- [ ] celery seeds
- [ ] hazelnuts
- [ ] sesame seeds

Condiments, Spreads and Sauces
- [ ] canola mayonnaise (such as Spectrum Organic®)

- ❑ Dijon mustard
- ❑ dressing, fat-free
- ❑ hoisin sauce
- ❑ honey
- ❑ honey mustard
- ❑ hot pepper sauce (such as Tabasco®)
- ❑ mango chutney
- ❑ mayonnaise, reduced fat
- ❑ peanut butter
- ❑ red wine vinegar
- ❑ relish, sweet pickle
- ❑ rice vinegar
- ❑ soy sauce, low-sodium
- ❑ strawberry spread, reduced-sugar (such as Smucker's®)
- ❑ vinegar, balsamic blend seasoned rice (such as Nakano®)
- ❑ vinegar, cider
- ❑ vinegar, white balsamic

Breads, Cereals and Pasta

- ❑ baked chips
- ❑ bagels
- ❑ bread, whole-grain
- ❑ brown rice
- ❑ cornflakes
- ❑ crackers, whole-wheat
- ❑ English muffin, whole-wheat
- ❑ farfalle (bow tie pasta)
- ❑ hamburger buns
- ❑ hoagie rolls
- ❑ panko (Japanese breadcrumbs)
- ❑ tortillas, corn
- ❑ tortillas, flour
- ❑ white rice
- ❑ wild rice

Canned Foods

- ❑ artichoke hearts
- ❑ capers

- ❑ chicken broth, fat-free
- ❑ garlic, minced
- ❑ pinto beans
- ❑ refried beans

Dairy Products

- ❑ butter
- ❑ cheddar cheese
- ❑ cheddar cheese, white
- ❑ Colby-Jack cheese
- ❑ feta cheese, reduced fat
- ❑ goat cheese
- ❑ Gruyère cheese
- ❑ margarine
- ❑ milk, fat-free
- ❑ mozzarella, part-skim
- ❑ Parmigiano-Reggiano cheese
- ❑ yogurt, fat-free vanilla
- ❑ yogurt, Greek style (such as Fage®)

Juices

- ❑ lemon juice
- ❑ lime juice
- ❑ orange juice

Frozen Foods

- ❑ corn kernels, frozen
- ❑ spinach, package
- ❑ sugar snap peas, package

Meat and Poultry

- ❑ chicken
- ❑ eggs
- ❑ flank steak
- ❑ ground round, extra-lean
- ❑ pork chops, bone-in center-cut
- ❑ pork tenderloins
- ❑ prosciutto
- ❑ salmon fillets
- ❑ shrimp
- ❑ trout fillets

First Week Meals and Recipes

DAY 1

Breakfast

Strawberry Jam Crumb Cake

1½ cups all-purpose flour
½ tsp. baking powder
¼ tsp. baking soda
¼ cup brown sugar, packed
¼ tsp. cinnamon, ground
⅛ tsp. salt
⅔ cup powdered sugar
¼ cup butter, softened
½ tsp. vanilla extract

2 tbsp. chilled butter, cut into
   small pieces
1 large egg
6 tbsp. fat-free milk
2 tbsp. lemon juice
¼ cup reduced-sugar strawberry
   spread (such as Smucker's®)
nonstick cooking spray

To prepare crumb topping, lightly spoon ¼ cup of the flour into a dry measuring cup and level with a knife. Combine the flour, brown sugar and cinnamon in a small bowl. Cut in 2 tablespoons chilled butter with a pastry blender or 2 knives until mixture resembles coarse meal and set aside. Preheat oven to 350° F. To prepare the cake, lightly coat an 8″ spring form pan with cooking spray and set aside. Lightly spoon the rest of the flour into dry measuring cups and level with a knife. Combine flour, baking powder, baking soda and salt in a small bowl and set aside. Combine the powdered sugar and ¼ cup butter in a large bowl, and beat with a mixer at medium speed until well blended (about 2 minutes). Add the vanilla extract and the egg and beat for 2 minutes. Combine the milk and lemon juice, add to the sugar mixture, and beat for 2 minutes. Add half of the flour mixture to sugar mixture and stir until smooth. Add the remaining flour mixture and stir just until combined. Spoon half of the batter into a prepared pan, spreading evenly, and top with the strawberry spread. Spoon the remaining batter over the strawberry layer, spreading evenly. Sprinkle the reserved crumb topping evenly over the batter. Bake at 350° F for 45 minutes or until a wooden pick inserted into the center comes out clean. Cool for 10 minutes in the pan on a wire rack, and then remove from the pan. Cool the cake completely on the wire rack. Serve with 6 oz. light fruit yogurt and a cup of orange juice. Serves 12.

Nutritional Information: 191 calories; 6g fat; 3g protein; 32g carbohydrate; 1g dietary fiber; 33mg cholesterol; 123mg sodium.

....

Lunch

Chicken Corn Chowder

1 tbsp. butter
6 green onions
2 tbsp. all-purpose flour
2 cups chicken breast, chopped
 and cooked
¼ tsp. salt
¼ tsp. black pepper, freshly ground

2 (10-oz.) packages frozen corn
 kernels, thawed and divided
1 (14-oz.) can fat-free chicken broth
2 cups fat-free milk
½ cup (2 oz.) cheddar cheese, pre-
 shredded

Melt butter in a Dutch oven over medium-high heat. Remove the green tops from the green onions, chop, and set aside. Thinly slice the white portion of each onion, add to a pan, and sauté for 2 minutes. Add flour and cook for 1 minute, stirring constantly with a whisk. Stir in chicken, salt, pepper, 1 package of corn and broth. Bring to a boil, and then reduce the heat and simmer for 5 minutes. While the mixture simmers, combine the remaining corn and milk in a blender and process until smooth. Add the milk mixture to the pan and simmer for 2 minutes or until thoroughly heated. Ladle 2 cups of the chowder into each of 4 soup bowls and sprinkle evenly with green onion tops. Top each serving with 2 tablespoons of the cheese. Serve with 6 whole-wheat crackers and a cup of fresh fruit. Serves 4.

Nutritional Information: 394 calories; 12g fat; 35.5g protein; 41g carbohydrate; 4.5g dietary fiber; 84mg cholesterol; 534mg sodium.

....

Dinner

Grilled Pork Tenderloin with Salsa

2 (1-lb.) pork tenderloins, trimmed
 and cut into ¾-inch slices
½ tsp. salt

½ tsp. black pepper, freshly ground
 and divided
1½ cups green tomato, diced

¼ cup flat-leaf parsley (fresh), chopped
3 tbsp. chives (fresh), thinly sliced
2 tbsp. lemon juice
2 tbsp. extra-virgin olive oil
1 tbsp. capers

1 tsp. oregano (fresh), chopped
1 tsp. thyme (fresh), chopped
1 tsp. sugar
1 garlic clove, minced
nonstick cooking spray

Prepare a grill on medium-high heat. Arrange the pork slices in a single layer between 2 sheets of heavy-duty plastic wrap and pound to ½-inch thickness using a meat mallet or small heavy skillet. Lightly coat the pork with non-stick cooking spray and sprinkle with salt and ¼ teaspoon of the pepper. Place the pork on a grill rack and grill for 2 minutes on each side or until done. Combine tomato, parsley, chives, lemon juice, olive oil, capers, oregano, thyme, sugar and garlic in a food processor and pulse until minced. Stir in the remaining ¼ teaspoon of the pepper and serve with the pork. Serve with 1 cup grilled vegetables and 4 oz. roasted potatoes. Serves 6.

Nutritional Information: 235 calories; 10g fat; 32g protein; 3g carbohydrate; 1g dietary fiber; 98mg cholesterol; 320 mg sodium.

DAY 2

Breakfast
½ toasted whole-wheat English muffin
1 tbsp. peanut butter
½ banana

1 cup skim milk

Top the English muffin with peanut butter and banana. Serve with skim milk. Serves 1.

Nutritional Information: 302 calories; 9g fat; 15g protein; 42g carbohydrate; 3g dietary fiber; 4mg cholesterol; 334mg sodium.

Lunch

Bow Tie Pasta with Fresh Asparagus
6 oz. farfalle (bow tie pasta), uncooked
2 cups grape tomatoes, halved

1 cup seedless green grapes, halved
⅓ cup fresh basil leaves, thinly sliced
2 tbsp. white balsamic vinegar

2 tbsp. shallots, chopped
2 tsp. capers
1 tsp. Dijon mustard
½ tsp. minced garlic
½ tsp. salt

¼ tsp. black pepper, freshly ground
4 tsp. extra-virgin olive oil
1 (4-oz.) package reduced-fat feta
  cheese, crumbled

Cook pasta according to package directions (omitting salt) and drain. Combine cooked pasta, tomatoes, grapes and basil in a large bowl. While the pasta cooks, combine vinegar, shallots, capers, Dijon mustard, minced garlic, salt and pepper in a small bowl, stirring with a whisk. Gradually add oil to the vinegar mixture, stirring constantly with a whisk. Drizzle vinaigrette over pasta mixture and toss well to coat. Add cheese and toss to combine. Next, combine 1 teaspoon of the extra-virgin olive oil, ¼ teaspoon of the salt and ⅛ teaspoon of the black pepper, and 1 pound trimmed asparagus. Heat a grill pan over medium-high heat. Coat the pan with nonstick cooking spray and add the asparagus mixture to the pan. Cook for 5 minutes or until tender, turning once. Serve with 1 cup mixed fruit salad. Serves 4.

Nutritional Information: 320 calories; 10g fat; 14g protein; 46g carbohydrate; 3g dietary fiber; 10mg cholesterol; 822mg sodium.

....

Dinner

Summer Beef Stir-fry

3 tbsp. rice vinegar, divided
2 tbsp. low-sodium soy sauce, divided
1 (1-lb.) flank steak, trimmed and
  thinly sliced across grain
2 tsp. sugar
2 tsp. hoisin sauce
¼ tsp. salt
¼ tsp. red pepper, crushed
2 tsp. toasted sesame oil, divided

1 cup onion, chopped
1 tsp. minced ginger
½ tsp. minced garlic
1 cup red bell pepper, chopped
½ cup carrots, matchstick-cut
1 (8-oz.) package sugar snap peas
1¼ cups green onions, chopped
1 cup white rice
1 tsp. sesame seeds, toasted

Combine 1 tablespoon of the vinegar, 1 tablespoon of the soy sauce and the beef in a large bowl. Combine the remaining 2 tablespoons vinegar, 1 tablespoon soy sauce, sugar, hoisin sauce, salt and crushed red pepper in a small bowl. Stir with a whisk. Heat a large nonstick skillet over medium-high heat. Add 1 teaspoon of the oil to the pan and swirl to coat. Add the beef mixture to the pan and stir-fry for 2 minutes or until done. Place beef mixture in a bowl. Heat the remaining 1 teaspoon oil in pan over medium-high heat. Add onion to pan and sauté for 1 minute. Add the ginger and garlic and sauté for 15 seconds. Stir in the bell pepper, carrot and peas and sauté for 3 minutes. Add the vinegar mixture and beef mixture to the pan and cook for 2 minutes or until thoroughly heated. Remove from the heat and stir in ½ cup of the green onions. Next, cook the white rice according to package directions (omitting salt). Remove from the heat and stir in ¾ cup of the chopped green onions and sesame seeds. Serve with a tossed salad with 1 tablespoon fat-free dressing. Serves 4.

Nutritional Information: 254 calories; 8g fat; 27g protein; 17g carbohydrate; 3g dietary fiber; 37mg cholesterol; 526mg sodium.

DAY 3

Breakfast

Herb and Goat Cheese Omelet

4 large eggs
1 tbsp. water
¼ tsp. black pepper, freshly ground
  and divided
⅛ tsp. salt
1 tsp. parsley (fresh), chopped
½ tsp. tarragon (fresh), chopped

¼ cup goat cheese, crumbled
2 tsp. extra-virgin olive oil, divided
½ cup zucchini, thinly sliced
½ cup red bell pepper, julienne-cut
dash of salt
1 tsp. chives (fresh), chopped

Combine eggs and 1 tablespoon water in a bowl, stirring with a whisk. Stir in ⅛ teaspoon of the pepper and ⅛ teaspoon of the salt. Combine parsley, tarragon and goat cheese in a small bowl. Heat 1 teaspoon of the extra-virgin olive oil in an 8″ nonstick skillet over medium heat. Add remaining ⅛ teaspoon pepper, zucchini, bell pepper and dash of salt to the pan and cook for 4 minutes or until tender. Remove the zucchini mixture from pan, cover and keep warm. Place ½ teaspoon of the olive oil in a skillet. Pour half of the egg mixture into pan and let the egg mixture set slightly (do not stir). Carefully loosen set edges of the omelet with a spatula, tipping the pan to pour uncooked egg to the sides. Continue this procedure for about 5 seconds or until almost no runny egg remains. Sprinkle half of the cheese mixture evenly over omelet and cook for 1 minute or until set. Slide the omelet onto a plate, folding it into thirds. Repeat this procedure with the remaining ½ teaspoon oil, egg mixture and goat cheese mixture. Sprinkle chives over omelets and serve with the zucchini mixture. Serve with 1 cup fresh juice. Serves 2.

Nutritional Information: 233 calories; 18g fat; 16g protein; 4g carbohydrate; 1g dietary fiber; 430mg cholesterol; 416mg sodium.

....

Lunch

Shrimp Po-Boys

⅓ cup plus 3 tbsp. reduced-fat mayonnaise
2 tbsp. sweet pickle relish
1 tbsp. shallots, chopped
1 tsp. capers, chopped
¼ tsp. hot pepper sauce (such as Tabasco®)
1 lb. large shrimp, peeled and deveined
1½ tsp. Cajun seasoning, salt-free

2 tsp. extra-virgin olive oil
4 (2½-oz.) hoagie rolls
½ cup romaine lettuce, shredded
8 thin tomato slices
4 thin red onion slices
4 cups green cabbage, shredded
1 cup carrots, shredded
1 tbsp. cider vinegar
¼ tsp. celery seeds

Combine the mayonnaise, relish, shallots, capers, hot pepper sauce and shrimp in a small bowl. Heat a large nonstick skillet over medium-high heat. Combine the shrimp and Cajun seasoning in a bowl and toss well. Add olive oil to pan and swirl to coat. Add the shrimp to the pan and cook for 2 minutes on each side or until done. Cut each roll in half horizontally. Top the bottom half of each roll with 2 tablespoons lettuce, 2 tomato slices, 1 onion slice, and one quarter of the shrimp. Spread the top half of each roll with about 2 tablespoons of the mayonnaise mixture and place on top of sandwich. Next, combine the green cabbage and shredded carrot in a large bowl. Combine 3 tablespoons of the reduced-fat mayonnaise with the cider vinegar and celery seeds in a small bowl. Add the mayonnaise mixture to the cabbage mixture and stir well. Serve with 1 ounce baked chips. Serves 4.

Nutritional Information: 401 calories; 31g protein; 44g carbohydrate; 3g dietary fiber; 172mg cholesterol; 944mg sodium.

Dinner

Spice-rubbed Chicken

1½ tsp. brown sugar
1¼ tsp. ground cumin
1 tsp. salt
½ tsp. black pepper, freshly ground
½ tsp. paprika

½ tsp. thyme, dried
½ tsp. chili powder
1 (4-lb.) chicken
nonstick cooking spray

Prepare a grill for indirect grilling. (If you are using a gas grill, heat one side to medium-high and leave one side with no heat. If you are using a charcoal grill, arrange hot coals on either side of charcoal grate, leaving an empty space in middle.) Combine sugar, cumin, salt, black pepper, paprika, thyme and chili power and set aside. Remove and discard the giblets and neck from the chicken and trim any excess fat. Place the chicken, breast side down, on a cutting surface. Cut the chicken in half lengthwise along the backbone, cutting to (but not through) the other side. Turn the chicken over and then, starting at neck cavity, loosen the skin from the breast and drumsticks by inserting your fingers and gently pushing between the skin and the meat. Rub the spice mixture under the skin and gently press to secure. Coat the grill rack with nonstick cooking spray and place the chicken, breast side down, on it over direct heat. Cover and cook the chicken for 7 minutes. Turn the chicken over and cook for an additional 7 minutes. Move the chicken over indirect heat, cover and cook 45 minutes or until a thermometer inserted in the meaty part of the thigh registers 165° F. Transfer the chicken to a cutting board, discard the skin, and let it sit for 10 minutes. Serve with 1 cup green beans, ½ cup mashed potatoes and a cup of fresh fruit. Serves 4.

Nutritional Information: 270 calories; 7g fat; 47g protein; 3g carbohydrate; 1g dietary fiber; 150mg cholesterol; 657mg sodium.

DAY 4

Breakfast

1 serving cornflakes (or other
   low-sugar cereal)

1 cup skim milk
1 banana, sliced

Nutritional Information: 347 calories; 1g fat; 12g protein; 76g carbohydrate; 4g dietary fiber; 4mg cholesterol; 574mg sodium.

Lunch

Grilled Chicken Salad

1½ cups 2% reduced-fat Greek-style
   yogurt (such as Fage®)
1 tbsp. canola oil
1 tbsp. ginger (fresh), grated and peeled
3 garlic cloves, minced
¾ tsp. salt, divided
½ tsp. red pepper, ground
1 cup green grapes, seedless
½ cup red onion, chopped

4 chicken breast halves, skinned and
   bone-in
½ cup mango chutney
⅓ cup celery, finely chopped
⅓ cup canola mayonnaise (such as
   Spectrum Organic®)
3 tbsp. lemon juice
nonstick cooking spray

Combine yogurt, canola oil, ginger and garlic cloves, stirring to combine. Stir in ¼ teaspoon of the salt and pepper. Place the yogurt mixture in a heavy-duty zip-top plastic bag. Add chicken to the bag and seal. Marinate in refrigerator for 2 hours, turning occasionally. Next, prepare a grill to medium-high heat. Remove the chicken from the bag and discard the marinade. Coat the grill rack with nonstick cooking spray and place the chicken, breast side down, on the rack. Grill for 10 minutes or until browned. Turn the chicken over; grill for 20 minutes or until a thermometer inserted inside the meaty part of the breast registers at 160° F. Remove the chicken from grill and let stand for 10 minutes. Remove the meat from the bones. Coarsely chop the chicken and place in a medium bowl. Sprinkle the chicken with the remaining ½ teaspoon salt. Add the remaining ¼ of the red pepper, grapes, red onion, mango chutney, celery, canola mayonnaise and lemon juice to the chicken mixture. Toss gently to combine. Chill for 30 minutes. Serves 5.

Nutritional Information: 430 calories; 19g fat; 29g protein; 35g carbohydrate; 1g dietary fiber; 68mg cholesterol; 718mg sodium.

Dinner

Grilled Pork Chops with Shallot Butter

8 (7-oz.) pork chops, bone-in and
   center-cut
1 tsp. salt, divided
¾ tsp. black pepper, freshly ground
2 tbsp. extra-virgin olive oil

2 tsp. chives (fresh), finely chopped
1 tsp. thyme (fresh), finely chopped
1 tsp. rosemary (fresh), finely
   chopped
3 garlic cloves, minced

2 tbsp. butter, softened   ¼ tsp. lemon rind, grated
2½ tsp. shallots, minced

Prepare a grill to medium-high heat. Sprinkle both sides of the pork evenly with ½ teaspoon salt and pepper. Combine oil, chives, thyme, rosemary and garlic, stirring well. Rub the oil mixture evenly over both sides of pork. Place the pork on grill rack and grill for 6 minutes on each side or until a thermometer inserted in the thickest part of the pork registers at 155° F. Remove the pork from grill and let stand 5 minutes. Sprinkle with remaining ½ teaspoon salt. Combine butter, shallots and lemon rind, stirring well. Spread about 1 teaspoon of the butter mixture over each pork chop and let the pork stand an additional 5 minutes. Serve with ⅔ cup steamed rice and *Artichoke and Eggplant Skewers* (see recipe below). Serves 8.

Nutritional Information: 208 calories; 12g fat; 23g protein; 1g carbohydrate; 0g dietary fiber; 68mg cholesterol; 360mg sodium.

Artichoke and Eggplant Skewers

3 tbsp. lemon juice
1 tsp. oregano (fresh), chopped
4 tsp. extra-virgin olive oil
2 garlic cloves, minced
6 frozen artichoke hearts, thawed
    and quartered
24 cherry tomatoes

24 (1-inch) cubes eggplant
    (about ¾ pound)
¼ tsp. salt
¼ tsp. black pepper, freshly ground
lemon wedges (optional)
nonstick cooking spray

Prepare a grill to medium-high heat. Combine lemon juice, oregano, olive oil and garlic in a small bowl and stir well with a whisk. Thread artichoke hearts, eggplant and tomatoes alternately onto each of 8 (10-inch) skewers. (Note that you can also use baby artichoke hearts, but you will need to blanch them first in boiling water with lemon juice for eight minutes or just until barely tender, and then quarter and arrange on skewers.) Coat a grill rack with nonstick cooking spray and place the skewers on it. Grill the skewers for 6 minutes or until tender, turning frequently. Place the skewers on a platter and brush with juice mixture. Sprinkle with salt and pepper. Serve with lemon wedges, if desired. Serves 8.

Nutritional Information: 45 calories; 3g fat; 1g protein; 6g carbohydrate; 2g dietary fiber; 0mg cholesterol; 80mg sodium.

DAY 5

Breakfast

Blueberry Pancakes

2¼ oz. all-purpose flour
   (about ½ cup)
½ cup whole-wheat flour
1 tbsp. sugar
1 tsp. baking powder
½ tsp. baking soda
⅛ tsp. salt
⅛ tsp. nutmeg, ground

¾ cup vanilla fat-free yogurt
2 tbsp. butter, melted
2 tsp. lemon juice
½ tsp. vanilla extract
2 large eggs, lightly beaten
1 cup fresh blueberries

Weigh or lightly spoon the all-purpose flour and whole-wheat flour into dry measuring cups and level with a knife. Combine the flours and sugar, baking powder, baking soda, salt and nutmeg in a large bowl, stirring well with a whisk. Combine the yogurt, butter, lemon juice, vanilla extract and eggs in a small bowl and add to the flour mixture, stirring until smooth. Pour about ¼ cup of the batter per pancake onto a hot nonstick griddle or a nonstick skillet. Top each pancake with 2 tablespoons blueberries. Cook for 2 minutes or until the tops are covered with bubbles and the edges look cooked. Carefully turn the pancakes over and cook for 2 minutes or until the bottoms are lightly browned. Serve with 1 cup skim milk. Serves 4.

Nutritional Information: 272 calories; 9g fat; 10g protein; 40g carbohydrate; 3g dietary fiber; 122mg cholesterol; 403mg sodium.

Lunch

Basil, Feta, Tomato Pizza

½ cup (2 oz.) part-skim mozzarella
   cheese, shredded
½ cup (2 oz.) reduced-fat feta cheese,
   finely crumbled
¼ cup (1 oz.) Parmigiano-Reggiano
   cheese, grated
1 tbsp. oregano (fresh), chopped
¼ tsp. salt

⅛ tsp. black pepper, freshly ground
10 (18″ x 14″) sheets frozen phyllo
   dough, thawed
2 cups plum tomatoes, thinly sliced
⅓ cup green onions, thinly sliced
¼ cup basil leaves (fresh)
nonstick cooking spray

Preheat the oven to 375° F. Combine mozzarella cheese, feta cheese, Parmi-giano-Reggiano cheese, oregano, salt and pepper in a bowl. Cut phyllo sheets in half crosswise. Working with 1 phyllo sheet half at a time (cover the re-maining dough to keep from drying), place the dough on a baking sheet coated with nonstick cooking spray. Coat the phyllo sheet with nonstick cooking spray. Repeat with 2 more layers of phyllo. Sprinkle with 2 table-spoons of the cheese mixture and repeat the layers 5 times, ending with 2 phyllo sheets. Coat the top phyllo sheet with nonstick cooking spray and sprinkle with 2 tablespoons of the cheese mixture. Pat the tomato slices with a paper towel. Arrange the tomato slices on top of the cheese, leaving a 1-inch border. Sprinkle with onions and the remaining 6 tablespoons of the cheese mixture. Bake at 375° F for 20 minutes or until golden brown. Sprinkle with basil leaves. Serve with a tossed green salad and fat-free dressing. Serves 6.

Nutritional Information: 195 calories; 7g fat; 9g protein; 25g carbohydrate; 2g dietary fiber; 11mg cholesterol; 526mg sodium.

....

Dinner

Grilled Cheese Burgers with Grilled Onions

1 tsp. extra-virgin olive oil	¼ tsp. garlic powder
4 cups red onion, vertically sliced	1 lb. extra-lean ground round
4 tsp. sugar	4 (½-oz.) slices white cheddar cheese
4 tsp. red wine vinegar	4 (1½-oz.) hamburger buns, toasted
¾ tsp. thyme (fresh), chopped	4 tsp. canola mayonnaise
¾ tsp. oregano (fresh), chopped	nonstick cooking spray
½ tsp. salt	

Prepare a grill on medium-high heat or use a heavy skillet for inside cook-ing. To prepare the grilled onions, heat a large nonstick skillet over medium-high heat. Add olive oil to the pan and swirl to coat. Add the red onion and sauté for 5 minutes. Reduce the heat to medium-low and stir in sugar, red wine vinegar and thyme. Cover and cook for 10 minutes or until the onion is tender, and then remove from the heat. To prepare the burgers, combine oregano, salt, garlic powder and beef in a bowl. Divide the mixture into 4 equal portions, shaping each into a ½-inch-thick patty. Coat the grill rack (or skillet) with nonstick cooking spray. Place the burgers on the rack and cook for 2 minutes or until browned. Turn the patties over, place 1 cheese slice on each patty, and cook for an additional 2 minutes or until done. Next, spread the cut sides of each bun with ½ teaspoon mayonnaise. Place 1 patty on the bottom half of each bun and top each with ¼ cup grilled onions and the bun top. Serve with 1 ounce baked chips and 1 cup fresh fruit with 1 tablespoon yogurt on top. Serves 4.

Nutritional Information: 395 calories; 14g fat; 34g protein; 36g carbohydrate; 3g dietary fiber; 75 mg cholesterol; 696mg sodium.

DAY 6

Breakfast

2 oz. bagel, toasted and topped with 1 tsp. light margarine

1 cup mixed fruit

Nutritional Information: 384 calories; 3g fat; 8g protein; 84g carbohydrate; 6g dietary fiber; 0mg cholesterol; 291mg sodium.

Lunch

Prosciutto, Lettuce and Tomato Sandwich

8 (1-oz.) slices 100% whole-grain bread
¼ cup canola mayonnaise
2 tbsp. basil (fresh), chopped
1 tsp. Dijon mustard

1 small garlic clove, minced
1 cup baby romaine lettuce leaves
8 (¼-inch-thick) slices of tomato
3 oz. prosciutto, sliced thin

Preheat a broiler. Arrange the bread slices in a single layer on a baking sheet. Broil the bread for 2 minutes on each side or until toasted. Combine the mayonnaise, basil, mustard and garlic in a bowl and spread the mixture evenly over 4 bread slices. Layer ¼ cup lettuce and 2 tomato slices over each serving and top evenly with prosciutto and remaining bread. Serve with fruit salad (combine 1 teaspoon fresh lime rind, 1 tablespoon fresh lime juice, 1 tablespoon honey and a dash of salt, and then drizzle over 4 cups mixed pre-cut fruit). Serves 4.

Nutritional Information: 243 calories; 9g fat; 12g protein; 28g carbohydrate; 4g dietary fiber; 19mg cholesterol; 808mg sodium.

....

Dinner
Hazelnut Crusted Trout

¼ cup panko (Japanese breadcrumbs)
2 tbsp. hazelnuts, toasted and finely chopped
½ tsp. salt
½ tsp. lemon rind, grated
½ tsp. thyme (fresh), minced

¼ tsp. black pepper, freshly ground
4 (6-oz.) trout fillets
lemon wedges (optional)
nonstick cooking spray

Preheat oven to 400° F. Combine panko, hazelnuts, salt, lemon rind, thyme and pepper in a small bowl. Line a baking sheet with foil and coat with nonstick cooking spray. Arrange the trout in a single layer on the baking sheet. Sprinkle the hazelnut mixture evenly over trout and bake at 400° F for 10 minutes or until the fish flakes easily when tested with a fork. Serve with lemon wedges, if desired. Serve with ⅔ cup wild rice, a tossed green salad with fat-free dressing, and *Marinated Summer Beans* (see recipe below). Serves 4.

Nutritional Information: 215 calories; 8g fat; 33g protein; 3g carbohydrate; 1g dietary fiber; 74mg cholesterol; 401mg sodium.

Marinated Summer Beans

3½ tsp. salt, divided
1 lb. green beans (fresh), trimmed
1 lb. wax beans (fresh), trimmed
3 tbsp. flat-leaf parsley (fresh), chopped
2 tbsp. extra-virgin olive oil

1 tbsp. lemon rind, grated
2 tbsp. lemon juice
1 tsp. red pepper, crushed
1 garlic clove, minced

Add 1 tablespoon salt and the green beans and wax beans to a large saucepan of boiling water. Cook for 6 minutes or until crisp-tender. Drain the beans and rinse with cold water. Combine the remaining ½ teaspoon salt and the parsley, olive oil, lemon rind, lemon juice, red pepper and garlic in a large bowl. Add the beans to the mixture and toss well. Chill for at least 1 hour, tossing occasionally. Serves 8.

Nutritional Information: 68 calories; 4g fat; 2g protein; 9g carbohydrate; 4g dietary fiber; 0mg cholesterol; 199mg sodium.

DAY 7

Breakfast

Easy Breakfast Burrito

1½ cups tomato, chopped
½ cup green onions, chopped
½ cup cilantro (fresh), chopped
2 tsp. lemon juice
¼ tsp. salt
¼ tsp. black pepper
dash of crushed red pepper
¼ tsp. chopped fresh oregano

⅛ tsp. salt
4 eggs, lightly beaten
nonstick cooking spray
¼ cup chopped onion
1 (2-oz.) can diced green chilies
4 (6-inch) corn tortillas
½ cup (2 oz.) shredded Colby-Jack
    cheese

To prepare the Pico de Gallo, combine tomato, green onions, cilantro, lemon juice, ⅛ teaspoon salt, ⅛ teaspoon black pepper and red pepper in a small bowl and set aside. To prepare the burritos, combine the chopped fresh oregano, ⅛ teaspoon salt, ⅛ teaspoon black pepper, eggs and red pepper in a small bowl, stirring well with a whisk. Heat a large nonstick skillet over medium heat. Coat the pan with nonstick cooking spray and then add the egg mixture, ¼ cup of the onions and the green chilies to the pan. Cook for 3 minutes or until the eggs are set, stirring frequently. Remove the pan from the heat and stir egg mixture well. Next, heat the corn tortillas according to package directions. Divide the egg mixture evenly among tortillas. Top each serving with 2 tablespoons shredded cheese and about ⅓ cup of the Pico de Gallo. Serve with 1 cup fruit juice. Serves 4.

Nutritional Information: 197 calories; 11g fat; 13g protein; 14g carbohydrate; 2g dietary fiber; 258mg cholesterol; 372mg sodium.

Lunch

Grilled Salmon & Spinach Salad

¼ cup orange juice
2 tbsp. extra-virgin olive oil
2 tbsp. balsamic blend seasoned rice
    vinegar (such as Nakano®)
½ tsp. honey mustard
2½ tsp. black pepper
1 garlic clove, minced

2 tbsp. lemon juice
4 (6-oz.) salmon fillets (about
    1-inch thick)
1 (6-oz.) package spinach
nonstick cooking spray
4 oranges, each peeled and cut
    into 6 slices

Preheat a grill to medium-high heat. To prepare the vinaigrette, combine olive oil, rice vinegar, honey mustard, ½ teaspoon black pepper and garlic clove in a large bowl. Stir the mixture well with a whisk. To prepare the salad, drizzle lemon juice over the salmon fillets and sprinkle with 2 teaspoons pepper. Coat the grill rack with nonstick cooking spray and place the fillets, skin side up, on the rack. Grill for 5 minutes on each side or until the fish flakes easily when tested with a fork. Remove the skin from fillets and discard. Add spinach to the vinaigrette in bowl and toss well. Place 2 cups of the spinach mixture on each of 4 serving plates and arrange 1 fillet and 6 orange slices on top of the greens. Serve with 1 cup fresh fruit salad. Serves 4.

Nutritional Information: 474 calories; 26g fat; 36g protein; 28g carbohydrate; 8g dietary fiber; 100mg cholesterol; 286mg sodium.

....

Dinner

Chicken Mushroom Quesadillas

1 tsp. extra-virgin olive oil
1 cup mushrooms, pre-sliced
½ cup onion, thinly sliced
⅛ tsp. salt
⅛ tsp. black pepper, freshly ground
1 tsp. garlic, minced

1 tbsp. sherry or red wine vinegar
2 (10-inch) fat-free flour tortillas
1 cup cooked chicken breast, shredded
1 cup arugula
½ cup (2 oz.) shredded Gruyère cheese
nonstick cooking spray

Heat a large nonstick skillet over medium-high heat. Add olive oil to the pan and swirl to coat. Add mushrooms, sliced onion, salt and pepper to the pan and sauté for 5 minutes. Stir in the garlic and sauté for 30 seconds. Add vinegar and cook for 30 seconds or until the liquid almost evaporates. Arrange half of the mushroom mixture over half of each tortilla. Top each tortilla with ½ cup chicken, ½ cup arugula and ¼ cup cheese. Fold the tortillas in half. Wipe the pan clean with a paper towel and heat over medium heat. Coat the pan with nonstick cooking spray and add the tortillas to the pan. Place a heavy skillet on top of tortillas and cook for 2 minutes on each side or until crisp. Top with the Pico de Gallo you made from breakfast or with salsa. Serve with ½ cup pinto beans or fat-free refried beans. Serves 1.

Nutritional Information: 270 calories; 9g fat; 25g protein; 20g carbohydrate; 3g dietary fiber; 64mg cholesterol; 391mg sodium.

Second Week Grocery List

Produce

- [ ] apples
- [ ] apricots, fresh
- [ ] apricots, dried
- [ ] asparagus
- [ ] blueberries
- [ ] carrots
- [ ] celery
- [ ] cilantro, fresh
- [ ] cremini mushrooms
- [ ] currants
- [ ] dried fruit
- [ ] golden raisins
- [ ] green beans
- [ ] green salad
- [ ] lemons
- [ ] onions
- [ ] oranges
- [ ] potatoes
- [ ] raisins
- [ ] red onions
- [ ] red pepper
- [ ] Roma tomatoes
- [ ] romaine lettuce
- [ ] scallions
- [ ] spinach, baby
- [ ] tangerines
- [ ] tarragon, fresh
- [ ] tomatoes

Baking Products

- [ ] butter
- [ ] canola oil
- [ ] flour, all-purpose
- [ ] flour, whole-wheat
- [ ] nonstick cooking spray
- [ ] oats, old-fashioned rolled
- [ ] olive oil, extra-virgin
- [ ] sugar
- [ ] vanilla extract

Spices

- [ ] basil, dried
- [ ] black pepper
- [ ] cumin
- [ ] mustard, dry
- [ ] garlic powder
- [ ] onion powder
- [ ] oregano
- [ ] paprika
- [ ] salt

Nuts/Seeds

- [ ] almonds
- [ ] celery seed
- [ ] flaxseeds
- [ ] pecans
- [ ] sesame seeds
- [ ] sunflower seeds
- [ ] walnuts

Condiments, Spreads and Sauces

- [ ] almond butter
- [ ] apricot preserves
- [ ] chili sauce
- [ ] cider vinegar
- [ ] Dijon mustard
- [ ] hoisin sauce

- ❏ honey
- ❏ horseradish
- ❏ hot sauce
- ❏ jam
- ❏ marinara sauce, low-sodium
- ❏ mayonnaise, light
- ❏ mustard, whole-grain
- ❏ peanut butter
- ❏ ranch dressing, light
- ❏ red wine vinegar
- ❏ soy sauce, reduced sodium

Breads, Cereals and Pasta
- ❏ baked chips
- ❏ bran flakes
- ❏ brown rice
- ❏ croutons, fat-free
- ❏ dinner rolls, whole-grain
- ❏ English muffins, whole-wheat
- ❏ French baguette
- ❏ French bread
- ❏ hamburger buns, whole-grain
- ❏ oatmeal
- ❏ panko (Japanese breadcrumbs)
- ❏ penne, whole-wheat
- ❏ pita bread
- ❏ puffed cereal, whole-grain
- ❏ rice
- ❏ rye bread
- ❏ saltine crackers
- ❏ sandwich rolls, whole-wheat

Canned Foods
- ❏ black beans

- ❏ chicken broth
- ❏ chives, minced
- ❏ ginger, minced
- ❏ jalapeño pepper, minced

Dairy Products
- ❏ cheddar cheese, reduced-fat
- ❏ feta cheese
- ❏ Gruyère cheese
- ❏ milk, lowfat
- ❏ milk, whole
- ❏ mozzarella cheese, part skim
- ❏ Parmesan cheese
- ❏ Ricotta cheese, low-fat
- ❏ yogurt, low-fat lemon
- ❏ yogurt, low-fat vanilla

Juices
- ❏ lemon juice
- ❏ lime juice
- ❏ orange juice

Frozen Foods
- ❏ French fries, baked
- ❏ waffles, whole-grain

Meat and Poultry
- ❏ chicken, diced
- ❏ chicken breasts
- ❏ chicken tenders
- ❏ crabmeat
- ❏ eggs
- ❏ pork tenderloin
- ❏ roast beef

Second Week Meals and Recipes

DAY 1

....

Breakfast

Blueberry Oatmeal

½ cup oatmeal, cooked   1 tsp. honey
½ cup blueberries

Add fresh blueberries to your oatmeal and drizzle honey on top. Serve with
1 cup low-fat milk.

Nutritional Information: 272 calories; 2g fat; 14g protein; 50g carbohydrate; 5g dietary fiber;
4mg cholesterol; 130mg sodium.

....

Lunch

Onion-smothered Chicken Sandwiches

1 tsp. extra-virgin olive oil   2 tbsp. Dijon mustard
2 cups onion, thinly sliced   1 tbsp. honey
¼ cup honey   ½ tsp. paprika
¼ cup cider vinegar   ⅛ tsp. salt
4 (4-oz.) chicken breast halves,   4 (1¼-oz.) slices rye bread, toasted
  skinned and boned   nonstick cooking spray

Heat the olive oil in a large nonstick skillet over medium-high heat. Add
onion and cook for 1 minute. Cover, reduce heat to medium, and cook for
another 6 minutes or until soft. Stir in ¼ cup honey and vinegar. Cook, uncovered, for 10 minutes, stirring occasionally. Set aside. While the onions are
cooking, place each chicken breast half between 2 sheets of heavy-duty plastic wrap and flatten to ½-inch thickness using a meat mallet or a rolling
pin. Combine mustard, 1 tablespoon honey, paprika and salt in a small
bowl. Brush half of the mustard mixture over the chicken. Heat a large grill
pan or skillet coated with nonstick cooking spray over medium-high heat.
Place the chicken, coated side down, in pan and cook for 4 minutes. Brush
the chicken with the remaining mustard mixture. Turn chicken over and
cook for 4 minutes or until done. Place 1 chicken breast on each toast slice

and top with 2 tablespoons of the onion mixture. Serve with 1 ounce baked chips and a tangerine. Serves 4.

Nutritional Information: 351 calories; 5g fat; 30g protein; 47g carbohydrate; 3g dietary fiber; 66mg cholesterol; 630mg sodium.

....

Dinner

Almond-crusted Chicken Fingers

canola oil
½ cup almonds, sliced
¼ cup whole-wheat flour
1½ tsp. paprika
½ tsp. garlic powder
½ tsp. dry mustard

¼ tsp. salt
⅛ tsp. pepper, freshly ground
1½ tsp. extra-virgin olive oil
4 egg whites
1 lb. chicken tenders

Preheat oven to 475° F. Set a wire rack on a foil-lined baking sheet and coat with nonstick cooking spray. Place almonds, flour, paprika, garlic powder, dry mustard, salt and pepper in a food processor and process until the almonds are finely chopped and the paprika is mixed throughout (about 1 minute). With the motor running, drizzle in the canola oil and process until combined. Transfer the mixture to a shallow dish. Whisk egg whites in a second shallow dish. Add chicken tenders to egg whites and turn to coat. Transfer each chicken tender to the almond mixture and turn to coat evenly. (Discard any remaining egg white and almond mixture.) Place the tenders on the prepared rack and coat with nonstick cooking spray. Turn and spray the other side and bake the tenders until golden brown, crispy and no longer pink in the center (about 20 to 25 minutes). Serve with 1 cup mashed potatoes, 1 cup steamed vegetables and a whole-grain dinner roll. Serves 4.

Nutritional Information: 147 calories; 4g fat; 21g protein; 4g carbohydrate; 1g dietary fiber; 49mg cholesterol; 214mg sodium.

DAY 2

....

Breakfast

Make-ahead Morning Meal

apple
2 oz. reduced-fat cheddar cheese

¼ cup walnuts
1 cup orange juice

Slice the cheese into cubes, bag your meal and go.

Nutritional Information: 386 calories; 18g fat; 20g protein; 3g dietary fiber; 12mg cholesterol; 350mg sodium.

....

Lunch

Deluxe Roast Beef Sandwich

1 tbsp. light mayonnaise
2 tsp. horseradish
2 tsp. chili sauce
2 (1-oz.) slices rye bread
1 romaine lettuce leaf

3 oz. deli roast beef, thinly sliced
2 (¼-inch-thick) slices tomato
1 (⅛-inch-thick) slice red onion,
    separated into rings

Combine mayonnaise, horseradish and chili sauce. Spread the mayonnaise mixture on one bread slice and top with lettuce leaf, roast beef, tomato slices, onion and the remaining bread slice. Serve with 1 ounce baked chips and an apple. Serves 1.

Nutritional Information: 412 calories; 13g fat; 25g protein; 51g carbohydrate; 6g dietary fiber; 5mg cholesterol; 1,122mg sodium.

....

Dinner

Crab Cake Burgers

1 lb. crabmeat
1 egg, lightly beaten
½ cup panko (Japanese breadcrumbs)
¼ cup light mayonnaise
2 tbsp. chives, minced
1 tbsp. Dijon mustard
1 tbsp. lemon juice

1 tsp. celery seed
1 tsp. onion powder
¼ tsp. pepper, freshly ground
4 dashes hot sauce
1 tbsp. extra-virgin olive oil
2 tsp. butter
6 whole-grain hamburger buns

Mix crab, egg, breadcrumbs, mayonnaise, chives, mustard, lemon juice, celery seed, onion powder, pepper and hot sauce in a large bowl. Form into 6 patties. Heat the olive oil and butter in a large nonstick skillet over medium heat until the butter stops foaming. Cook the patties until golden brown (about 4 minutes per side). Serve with one ounce baked French fries. Serves 6.

Nutritional Information: 363 calories; 8g fat; 16g protein; 6g carbohydrate; 0g dietary fiber; 86mg cholesterol; 350mg sodium.

DAY 3

Breakfast

Peanut Butter Waffle

1 tbsp. peanut butter
2 whole-grain frozen waffles

1 tbsp. raisins

Toast the waffles, spread with peanut butter and sprinkle with raisins. Serve with 1 cup low-fat milk.

Nutritional Information: 388 calories; 12g fat; 12g protein; 64g carbohydrate; 0g dietary fiber; 0mg cholesterol; 1mg sodium.

Lunch

Super Quick Black Bean Soup

½ cup red onion, chopped
2 tsp. extra-virgin olive oil
1 tsp. garlic, minced
¾ tsp. oregano
¾ tsp. cumin

1 can (15 oz.) black beans, drained
  and rinsed
2 cups chicken broth
1 tbsp. feta cheese
cilantro (optional)

In a large saucepan, combine onion, oil, garlic, oregano, cumin and salt. Cook, stirring, over medium heat until softened (about 3 minutes). Stir in beans and broth. Reduce heat to medium-low and cook, stirring occasionally, for 10 minutes. Mash some beans against the side of the pan. Serve sprinkled with feta cheese and cilantro (optional). Serve with 6 saltine crackers and 1 cup baby carrots with 2 tablespoons light ranch dressing. Serves 2.

Nutritional Information: 236 calories; 8g fat; 15g protein; 36g carbohydrates; 11g dietary fiber; 4mg cholesterol; 563mg sodium.

Dinner

Super Fast Stir-fry

1 tsp. extra-virgin olive oil
½ cup onion, diced
½ cup red pepper, diced

1 egg
1 tbsp. reduced-sodium soy sauce
dash of hot sauce

1 cup chicken, precooked and diced   2 scallions, chopped
1 cup brown rice, cooked

Heat the olive oil in a nonstick skillet over medium heat. Add the onion and red pepper and sauté for 3 to 5 minutes, until the onion softens. Add the egg, stirring frequently. Cook for 2 to 4 minutes more, until the egg firms up. Add the soy sauce, hot sauce, chicken, rice and scallions. Stir and cook for about 3 minutes more, until all the ingredients are well blended. Serves 2.

Nutritional Information: 333 calories; 8g fat; 32g protein; 32g carbohydrate; 4g dietary fiber; 165mg cholesterol; 849mg sodium.

DAY 4

Breakfast
Morning Pizza
2 (½-inch) slices French baguette   1 tsp. extra-virgin olive oil
3 tbsp. low-fat Ricotta cheese   dash of salt
1 Roma tomato, sliced   dash of pepper

Layer baguette slices, ricotta cheese and tomato and drizzle with olive oil. Season with salt and pepper and broil in oven for 3 to 4 minutes until hot and toasty. Serve with 1 cup orange juice. Serves 1.

Nutritional Information: 277 calories; 12g fat; 14g protein; 28g carbohydrate; 3g dietary fiber; 26mg cholesterol; 321mg sodium.

Lunch
Cheddar-apple Melt
1 whole-wheat English muffin,   4 apple slices, cut thin
  toasted   2 slices reduced-fat Cheddar
2 tsp. jam (or chutney)   cheese

Top the English muffin with jam (or chutney), apple and cheese. Toast in a toaster oven or under a broiler until the cheese is melted. Serve with one cup of mixed fruit with low-fat yogurt for dipping. Serves 1.

Nutritional Information: 253 calories; 5g fat; 20g protein; 33g carbohydrate; 1g dietary fiber; 12mg cholesterol; 769mg sodium.

....

Dinner

Apricot Pork Tenderloin

1½ cups chopped apricots
⅓ cup apricot preserves
1 tbsp. hoisin sauce
1 tbsp. reduced-sodium soy sauce
dash of salt

dash of pepper
1 lb. pork tenderloin, cut into
   1-inch pieces
2 tsp. extra-virgin olive oil

Combine the apricots, preserves, hoisin sauce and soy sauce in a small bowl. Season the pork with salt and pepper. Heat the olive oil in a large skillet over medium-high heat and add the pork. Cook, stirring, until lightly browned (about 5 minutes). Stir in the apricot mixture. Bring to a boil, reduce the heat to low, cover and simmer for another 10 minutes, or until the pork is cooked through and the sauce is thick. Serve with ½ cup cooked brown rice and one serving of *Creamy Green Beans* (see recipe below). Serves 4.

Nutritional Information: 249 calories; 5g fat; 25g protein; 26g carbohydrate; 2g dietary fiber; 73mg cholesterol; 560mg sodium.

Creamy Green Beans

1 lb. fresh green beans, trimmed and
   cut into 1-inch pieces
3 tbsp. light mayonnaise

2 tsp. Dijon mustard
⅛ tsp. salt

Place beans in a steamer basket and steam over 2 inches of boiling water until tender (about 5 to 7 minutes). Whisk mayonnaise, mustard and salt in a medium bowl. Add the beans and toss to coat.

Nutritional Information: 57 calories; 2g fat; 2g protein; 10g carbohydrate; 4g dietary fiber; 0mg cholesterol; 240mg sodium.

DAY 5

....

Breakfast

Cereal Sundae to Go

1½ cups bran flakes
8 oz. lemon or vanilla low-fat yogurt

¼ cup dried fruit
1 tbsp. pecans, chopped

Mix all in a to-go container and go.

Nutritional Information: 395 calories; 6g fat; 11g protein; 91g carbohydrate; 13g dietary fiber; 0mg cholesterol; 529mg sodium.

....

Lunch

McDonald's Fast Food to Go

McPremium Grilled Chicken   1 orange
  Classic Sandwich®

Nutritional Information: 370 calories; 5g fat; 32 protein; 50g carbohydrate; 3g dietary fiber; 65mg cholesterol; 1,110mg sodium.

....

Dinner

Creamy Asparagus Pasta

8 oz. whole-wheat penne pasta
1 bunch asparagus, trimmed and cut
  into ¾-inch pieces
1½ cups whole milk
4 tsp. whole-grain mustard
4 tsp. all-purpose flour
½ tsp. salt
½ tsp. pepper, freshly ground
2 tsp. extra-virgin olive oil

3 tbsp. garlic, minced
2 tsp. tarragon (fresh), minced
  (or ½ tsp. dried)
1 tsp. lemon zest, freshly grated
2 tsp. lemon juice
½ cup Parmesan cheese, grated
  and divided

Bring a large pot of water to a boil. Add pasta and cook for 3 minutes less than the package directions. Add asparagus and continue cooking until the pasta and asparagus are just tender (about 3 minutes more). Drain the pasta and return to the pot. Whisk the milk, mustard, flour, salt and pepper in a medium bowl. Heat the olive oil in a medium saucepan over medium-high heat. Add garlic and cook, stirring, until fragrant and lightly browned (about 30 seconds to 1 minute). Whisk in the milk mixture and bring to a simmer, stirring constantly, and cook until thickened (about 1 to 2 minutes). Stir in tarragon, lemon zest and juice, and then stir the sauce into the pasta-asparagus mixture. Cook over medium-high heat, stirring, until the sauce is thick, creamy and coats the pasta (about 1 to 2 minutes). Stir in ¼ cup of the Parmesan cheese. Divide the pasta among 4 bowls and top with the remaining ¼ cup Parmesan cheese. Serve with 2-inch slice of French bread and mixed green salad with light ranch dressing. Serves 4.

Nutritional Information: 359 calories; 10g fat; 18g protein; 55g carbohydrate; 7g dietary fiber; 18mg cholesterol; 602mg sodium.

DAY 6

Breakfast

Mushroom, Tomato and Gruyère Breakfast Casserole

4 whole-wheat English muffins, split
1 tbsp. extra-virgin olive oil
2 medium tomatoes, chopped
1 lb. cremini or button mushrooms, trimmed and sliced
dash of salt
dash of pepper

8 eggs
½ cup lowfat milk
½ tsp. garlic powder
½ tsp. onion powder
2 tsp. dried basil
1 cup Gruyère cheese, grated

Arrange the English muffin halves in the bottom of a greased 9″ x 13″ baking dish, cutting them to fit if necessary, and set aside. Heat the olive oil in a large skillet over medium heat. Add tomatoes, mushrooms and salt and pepper. Cook, stirring occasionally, until tender and liquid is thickened (about 8 to 10 minutes). Spoon the tomato mixture over the top of the English muffins, distributing it evenly, and set aside to let cool. In a large bowl, whisk together eggs, milk, garlic powder, onion powder, salt and pepper. Pour evenly over tomato mixture and then sprinkle with basil. Cover and chill overnight. Set the dish aside at room temperature for 1 hour. Next, preheat an oven to 350° F. Sprinkle casserole with cheese and bake, uncovered, until puffed, cooked through and cheese is golden brown (about 45 to 50 minutes). Serves 8.

Nutritional Information: 240 calories; 12g fat; 15g protein; 19g carbohydrate; 3g dietary fiber; 225mg cholesterol; 430mg sodium.

Lunch

Crab Salad-stuffed Pitas

1 tbsp. red wine vinegar
1 tbsp. extra-virgin olive oil

1 tsp. lime juice
dash of pepper, freshly ground

1 tsp. fresh ginger, minced
7 oz. crab meat, cooked and drained
½ cup celery hearts with leaves, finely
chopped
2 tbsp. red onion, minced
1 tbsp. cilantro (fresh), chopped

1 tsp. jalapeño pepper, minced
2 (6-inch) pita breads, warmed and
cut in half crosswise
2 large romaine lettuce leaves,
torn in half

Whisk the vinegar, oil, lime juice and pepper in a medium bowl. Add ginger, crab, celery, onion, cilantro and jalapeño and toss well. Line the pita halves with lettuce and fill with crab salad. Serve with one cup mixed fruit. Serves 2.

Nutritional Information: 339 calories: 10g fat; 28g protein; 38g carbohydrate; 6g dietary fiber; 70mg cholesterol; 728mg sodium.

Dinner

KFC Dinner to Go
Honey BBQ Sandwich®

3″ corn on the cob

Nutritional Information: 360 calories; 9g fat; 22g protein; 40g carbohydrate; 3g dietary fiber; 60mg cholesterol; 780mg sodium.

DAY 7

Breakfast

Almond-honey Power Bar
1 cup old-fashioned rolled oats
¼ cup almonds, slivered
¼ cup sunflower seeds
1 tbsp. flaxseeds (preferably golden)
1 tbsp. sesame seeds
1 cup whole-grain puffed cereal,
unsweetened
⅓ cup currants
⅓ cup dried apricots, chopped

⅓ cup golden raisins, chopped
¼ cup creamy almond butter
(or peanut butter)
¼ cup sugar
¼ cup honey
½ tsp. vanilla extract
⅛ tsp. salt
nonstick cooking spray

Preheat oven to 350° F. Coat an 8-inch square pan with nonstick cooking spray. Spread oats, almonds, sunflower seeds, flaxseeds and sesame seeds on a large, rimmed baking sheet. Bake until the oats are lightly toasted and the nuts are fragrant, shaking the pan halfway through (about 10 minutes). Transfer to a large bowl and add cereal, currants, apricots and raisins. Toss to combine. Next, combine almond butter, sugar, honey, vanilla and salt in a small saucepan. Heat over medium-low heat, stirring frequently, until the mixture bubbles lightly (about 2 to 5 minutes). Immediately pour the almond butter mixture over the dry ingredients and mix with a spoon or spatula until no dry spots remain. Transfer the mixture to the prepared pan. Lightly coat your hands with nonstick cooking spray and press the mixture down firmly to make an even layer (wait until the mixture cools slightly if necessary). Refrigerate until firm (about 30 minutes) amd cut into 8 bars. Store in airtight container for up to one week or freeze for one month. Serve with 1 cup low-fat milk.

Nutritional Information: 244 calories; 10g fat; 5g protein; 38g carbohydrate; 3g dietary fiber; 0mg cholesterol; 74mg sodium.

....

Lunch

Chicken Parmesan Sub

½ cup all-purpose flour
½ tsp. salt
½ tsp. pepper, freshly ground
1 lb. chicken breasts, boneless and skinless (2 large breasts cut into 4 portions or 4 small breasts)
4 tsp. extra-virgin olive oil, divided
2 (6-oz.) bags baby spinach

1 cup marinara sauce, preferably low-sodium
¼ cup Parmesan cheese, grated
½ cup part-skim mozzarella cheese, shredded
4 whole-wheat sandwich rolls, toasted

Position an oven rack in the top position and preheat broiler. Combine flour, salt and pepper in a shallow dish. Place the chicken between 2 large pieces of plastic wrap. Pound with the smooth side of a meat mallet or a heavy saucepan until the chicken is an even ¼-inch thickness. Dip the chicken in the flour mixture and turn to coat. Heat 2 teaspoons olive oil in a large nonstick skillet over medium-high heat. Add the spinach and cook, stirring often, until wilted (2 to 3 minutes). Transfer to a small bowl. Add 1 teaspoon olive oil to the pan. Add half the chicken and cook until golden, about 1 to 2 minutes per side. Transfer to a large baking sheet. Repeat with the remaining 1 teaspoon oil and chicken and then transfer to the baking sheet. Top each piece of chicken with the wilted spinach, marinara sauce and Parmesan cheese. Sprinkle with mozzarella and broil until the cheese is melted and the chicken is cooked through (about 3 minutes). Place on rolls and serve with 1 cup baby carrots with light ranch dressing. Serves 4.

Nutritional Information: 467 calories; 13g fat; 42g protein; 48g carbohydrate; 5g dietary fiber; 78mg cholesterol; 762mg sodium.

Dinner

Grilled Chicken Caesar Salad

1 lb. chicken breasts, boneless, skinless and trimmed of fat
1 tsp. canola oil
¼ tsp. salt
dash of pepper, freshly ground

8 cups washed, dried and torn romaine lettuce
1 cup fat-free croutons
½ cup Caesar salad dressing
½ cup Parmesan cheese curls

Prepare a grill or preheat a broiler. Rub the chicken with canola oil and season with salt and pepper. Grill or broil the chicken until browned and no trace of pink remains in the center (about 3 to 4 minutes per side). Combine the lettuce and croutons in a large bowl. Toss with Caesar salad dressing and divide among 4 plates. Cut the chicken into ½-inch slices and fan over the salad. Top with Parmesan cheese curls. Serve with lemon wedges. Serves 4.

Nutritional Information: 278 calories; 6g fat; 34g protein; 14g carbohydrate; 1g dietary fiber; 74mg cholesterol; 662mg sodium.

SNACK RECIPES

Basil Parmesan Dip with Pita Chips

4 (6-inch) pitas
½ tsp. black pepper, freshly ground and divided
¼ tsp. salt
1 cup basil leaves, lightly packed
¾ cup reduced-fat sour cream

¾ cup Parmigiano-Reggiano cheese, finely grated
2 tsp. lemon juice
1 garlic clove, minced
basil sprigs (optional)
nonstick cooking spray

Preheat oven to 375° F. Split the pitas and cut each half into 8 wedges. Place the wedges on a baking sheet. Coat with nonstick cooking spray and sprinkle with ¼ teaspoon of the pepper and salt. Bake at 375° F for 12 minutes or until crisp. Combine the remaining ¼ teaspoon pepper, basil leaves,

Parmigiano-Reggiano cheese, sour cream, lemon juice and garlic in a blender or food processor and process until smooth. Scrape into a serving bowl using a rubber spatula and garnish with basil sprigs, if desired. Serve with pita chips. Serves 8.

Nutritional Information: 153 calories; 5g fat; 7g protein; 19g carbohydrate: 1g dietary fiber; 18mg cholesterol; 362mg sodium.

Spiced Pecans

1 large egg white
1 tsp. water
2 cups pecan halves
½ cup sugar
1 tsp. cinnamon, ground

½ tsp. allspice, ground
⅛ tsp. black pepper, freshly
 ground
nonstick cooking spray

Preheat an oven to 250° F. Combine the egg white and 1 teaspoon of the water in a small bowl, stirring with a whisk until it turns frothy. Stir in the pecans and add sugar, cinnamon, allspice and black pepper, tossing to coat. Spread the nut mixture on a jelly-roll pan coated with nonstick cooking spray. Bake at 250° F for 45 minutes or until dry, stirring once. Cool completely. Serves 16.

Nutritional Information: 119 calories; 10g fat; 2g protein; 8g carbohydrate; 1g dietary fiber; 0mg cholesterol; 4mg sodium.

Basil Lemonade

4 cups water
½ cup lemon juice
½ cup basil leaves, loosely packed

6 tbsp. sugar
4 cups ice
4 basil sprigs

Combine 4 cups water and the lemon juice in a large bowl. Place ½ cup of the basil and the sugar in a mortar and pound with pestle until a paste forms (or use a food processor with ½ cup water). Add the sugar mixture to the juice mixture and stir until the sugar dissolves. Strain the mixture through a sieve over a bowl and discard the solids. Place 1 cup ice in each of 4 glasses. Pour about 1 cup of the lemonade into each glass and garnish with 1 basil sprig. Serves 4.

Nutritional Information: 82 calories; 0g fat; 0g protein; 22g carbohydrate; 0g dietary fiber; 0mg cholesterol; 5mg sodium.

Summer Biscotti

6 tbsp. sugar
2 tbsp. butter, softened
1½ tsp. lemon rind, grated
¼ tsp. vanilla extract
1 large egg
1 large egg white
¾ tsp. baking powder

4½ oz. all-purpose flour
(about 1 cup)
⅛ tsp. salt
½ cup white chocolate chips, divided
⅓ cup pecans, chopped
1 tbsp. fat-free half-and-half
nonstick cooking spray

Place sugar, butter, lemon rind and vanilla extract in a large bowl and beat with a mixer at high speed for 2 minutes until well blended. Add egg and egg white, one at a time, beating well after each addition. Weigh or lightly spoon the flour into a dry measuring cup and level with a knife. Combine the flour, baking powder and salt in a small bowl, stirring well with a whisk. Add the flour mixture to the sugar mixture, stirring until blended. Stir in ¼ cup of the chips and pecans (the dough will be sticky). Cover and chill for 30 minutes. Next, preheat oven to 325° F. Turn the dough out onto a heavily floured surface. With floured hands, shape the dough into a 9″ x 4″ log and pat to ½-inch thickness. Place the log on a baking sheet coated with nonstick cooking spray. Bake at 325° F for 30 minutes. Remove the log from pan and cool for 10 minutes on a wire rack. Cut the log crosswise into 18 (½-inch thick) slices. Place, cut sides down, on a baking sheet. Bake at 325° F for 15 minutes or until lightly browned. Cool completely on the wire rack. Place the remaining ¼ cup white chocolate chips in a glass measure and microwave on high for 30 seconds or just until melted. Add fat-free half-and-half and stir until smooth. Drizzle the mixture over the biscotti. Serves 18.

Nutritional Information: 95 calories; 4g fat; 2g protein; 13g carbohydrate; 1g dietary fiber; 15mg cholesterol; 50mg sodium.

Minted Watermelon Frozen Pops

¼ cup plus 6 tbsp. sugar
¾ cup water
¼ cup mint (fresh), coarsely chopped
2 cups (½-inch) seeded watermelon,
cubed

1 tbsp. lime juice
⅔ cup lemon juice
⅓ cup orange juice
¼ tsp. orange extract

To prepare the watermelon layer, combine ¼ cup of the sugar and ¼ cup of the water in a small saucepan over medium-high heat. Bring to a boil and cook for 30 seconds, stirring until the sugar dissolves. Stir in mint, and then cover and let stand for 30 minutes. Strain through a sieve into a bowl. Place the watermelon in a blender and process until smooth. Strain the puree through a sieve into bowl with mint syrup and press with the back of a spoon to extract the juice. Discard the solids. Next, stir in the lime juice, and then cover and chill for 1 hour. Pour about 2½ tablespoons of the watermelon mixture into each of 8 ice pop molds. Freeze for 1½ hours or until almost set. Arrange 1 wooden stick into mixture, being careful not to push through to bottom of the mold. Return to the freezer and freeze for 1 hour or until frozen. To prepare the lemon layer, combine 6 tablespoons of the sugar and ½ cup of the water in a small saucepan over medium-high heat. Bring to a boil and cook for 30 seconds, stirring until the sugar dissolves. Pour into a bowl and stir in the lemon juice, orange juice and extract. Cool for 15 minutes, and then cover and chill for at least 1 hour. Remove the molds from the freezer and pour about 3 tablespoons of the lemon mixture over the frozen watermelon mixture in each mold. Freeze for 2 hours or until completely frozen. Serves 8.

Nutritional Information: 82 calories; 0g fat; 0g protein; 22g carbohydrate; 0g dietary fiber; 0mg cholesterol; 3mg sodium.

DESSERT RECIPES

Banana Oatmeal Chocolate Chip Cookies

½ cup ripe banana, mashed
½ cup brown sugar, packed
¼ cup butter, softened
¼ cup granulated sugar
1 tsp. vanilla extract
1 large egg
2 cups old-fashioned oats

5½ oz. all-purpose flour (about 1¼ cups)
1 tsp. baking soda
½ tsp. salt
½ cup semisweet chocolate chips
nonstick cooking spray

Preheat oven to 350° F. Combine banana, brown sugar, butter, sugar and vanilla extract in a large bowl. Beat with a mixer at medium speed until smooth. Add the egg and beat well. Weigh or lightly spoon the flour into dry measuring cups and level with a knife. Combine flour, oats, baking soda and salt in a medium bowl, stirring with a whisk. Add the flour mixture to the banana mixture in bowl and beat with a mixer at medium speed until well blended. Stir in the chocolate chips. Next, drop the batter by heaping tablespoonfuls 2 inches apart onto baking sheets coated with nonstick cooking spray. Bake at 350° F for 18 minutes or until golden brown. Cool on pans for 2 minutes. Remove the cookies from pans and cool completely on wire racks. Serves 24.

Nutritional Information: 115 calories; 4g fat; 2g protein; 19g carbohydrate; 1g dietary fiber; 14mg cholesterol; 121mg sodium.

Orange Chiffon Cake

1½ tsp. baking powder
½ tsp. salt
8 oz. granulated sugar, divided
6 oz. cake flour, sifted
1 tbsp. orange rind, grated
½ cup orange juice
1 tbsp. lemon rind, grated

5 tbsp. canola oil
1½ tsp. vanilla extract
3 large egg yolks
8 large egg whites
¾ tsp. cream of tartar
2 tsp. powdered sugar

Preheat oven to 325° F. Combine baking powder, salt, 7 ounces of the sugar, and the flour in a large bowl, stirring with a whisk until mixture is well combined. Combine orange rind, orange juice, lemon rind, canola oil, vanilla extract and egg yolks in a medium bowl, stirring with a whisk. Add the rind mixture to the flour mixture, stirring until smooth. Place the egg whites in a large bowl and beat with a mixer at high speed until foamy. Add cream of tartar and beat until soft peaks form. Gradually add the remaining 1 ounce sugar, beating until stiff peaks form. Next, gently stir one-fourth of the egg white mixture into the flour mixture, and then gently fold in the remaining egg white mixture. Spoon the batter into an ungreased 10-inch tube pan, spreading evenly. Break any air pockets by cutting through the batter with a knife. Bake at 325° F for 45 minutes or until the cake springs back when lightly touched. Invert the pan and cool completely. Loosen the cake from sides of pan using a narrow metal spatula. Invert the cake onto a plate and sift powdered sugar over top of cake. Serves 16.

Nutritional Information: 158 calories; 5g fat; 3g protein; 24g carbohydrate; 0g dietary fiber; 38mg cholesterol; 149mg sodium.

Black and White Angel Food Cake

1 cup cake flour (about 4 oz.)
1½ cups granulated sugar, divided

½ tsp. cream of tartar
¼ tsp. salt

12 large egg whites
1 tsp. lemon juice
½ tsp. vanilla extract
2¾ tbsp. unsweetened dark cocoa
(such as Hershey's Special Dark®)

1½ cups powdered sugar
2 tbsp. light cream cheese, softened
1 tbsp. lowfat milk
1 tsp. vanilla extract
sliced strawberries (optional)

Preheat oven to 325° F. To prepare the cake, lightly spoon the flour into a dry measuring cup and level with a knife. Combine the flour and ¾ cup granulated sugar, stirring with a whisk, and set aside. Place cream of tartar, salt and egg whites in a large bowl and beat with a mixer at high speed until foamy. Add the remaining ¾ cup granulated sugar, 1 tablespoon at a time, beating until stiff peaks form. Beat in juice and ½ teaspoon vanilla. Sift the flour mixture over the egg white mixture, ¼ cup at a time, folding in after each addition. Spoon half of the batter into an ungreased 10-inch tube pan, spreading evenly. Break any air pockets by cutting through the batter with a knife. Sift 2 tablespoons cocoa over the remaining batter and fold in. Spoon cocoa batter evenly over the top of the vanilla batter, breaking air pockets by cutting through cocoa layer with a knife. Bake at 325° F for 55 minutes or until cake springs back when lightly touched. Invert the pan and cool completely. Loosen the cake from the sides of the pan using a narrow metal spatula. Invert the cake onto a plate. To prepare the glaze, place powdered sugar, cream cheese, milk and 1 teaspoon vanilla in a medium bowl. Beat with a mixer at medium speed until smooth. Drizzle half of the glaze over the cake. Add ¾ teaspoon cocoa to remaining glaze and stir well to combine. Drizzle the cocoa glaze over the cake. Refrigerate for 5 minutes or until the glaze is set. Garnish with strawberries, if desired. Serves 12.

Nutritional Information: 210 calories; 1g fat; 5g protein; 47g carbohydrate; 1g dietary fiber; 1mg cholesterol; 111mg sodium.

Fresh Fig Tart

1½ cups plus 2 tbsp. all-purpose
flour
¼ cup plus 2 tbsp. sugar
½ tsp. cinnamon, ground
⅛ tsp. salt
6 tbsp. butter, chilled and cut into
small pieces
1 tsp. vanilla extract

1 large egg
2 lbs. firm ripe black mission figs,
trimmed
2 tbsp. honey
¾ cup 2% reduced-fat Greek-style
yogurt
nonstick cooking spray

Preheat oven to 400° F. To prepare crust, coat a 9-inch round removable-bottom tart pan with cooking spray and set aside. Weigh or lightly spoon 6¾ ounces flour into dry measuring cups and level with a knife. Combine the flour, 2 tablespoons sugar, cinnamon and salt in a food processor and pulse to combine. With the processor on, gradually add butter through food chute, processing until the mixture resembles wet sand. Combine vanilla extract and egg in a small bowl and stir with a whisk. With the processor on, gradually add the egg mixture, processing until dough forms. Turn the dough out into a prepared pan and gently press into bottom and up sides of pan. Chill for 30 minutes. To prepare the filling, thinly slice figs to measure 1½ cups. Cut the remaining figs into ½-inch pieces (about 5 cups). Combine the fig pieces, ¼ cup sugar and 2 tablespoons flour, tossing to coat the figs. Spoon the fig mixture into the prepared crust. Bake at 400° F for 20 minutes, and then reduce the oven temperature to 350° F (do not remove tart from oven). Bake an additional 25 minutes or until bubbly. Remove from the oven and arrange fig slices over the top of tart. Next, place the honey in a microwave-safe bowl. Microwave on high for 1 minute, and then brush over the fig slices. Cool the tart slightly on a wire rack and serve warm with yogurt. Serves 12.

Nutritional Information: 224 calories; 7g fat; 4g protein; 37g carbohydrate; 3g dietary fiber; 34mg cholesterol; 77mg sodium.

Member Survey

Please answer the following questions to help your leader plan your First Place 4 Health meetings so that your needs might be met in this session. Give this form to your leader at the first group meeting.

Name _____ Birth date _____

Please list those who live in your household.

Name	Relationship	Age

What church do you attend? _____

Are you interested in receiving more information about our church?

      Yes   No

Occupation _____

What talent or area of expertise would you be willing to share with our class?

_____

Why did you join First Place 4 Health?

_____

With notice, would you be willing to lead a Bible study discussion one week?

      Yes   No

Are you comfortable praying out loud? _____

If the assistant leader were absent, would you be willing to assist in weighing in members and possibly evaluating the Live It Trackers?

      Yes   No

Any other comments:

_____

_____

Personal Weight and Measurement Record

Week	Weight	+ or -	Goal this Session	Pounds to goal
1				
2				
3				
4				
5				
6				

Beginning Measurements

Waist _____ Hips _____ Thighs _____ Chest _____

Ending Measurements

Waist _____ Hips _____ Thighs _____ Chest _____

First Place 4 Health
Prayer Partner

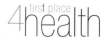

I will instruct you and teach you in the way you should go;
I will counsel you and watch over you.

PSALM 32:8

Date: _____

Name: _____

Home Phone: (_____) _____

Work Phone: (_____) _____

Email: _____

Personal Prayer Concerns:

_____

_____

_____

_____

_____

_____

_____

This form is for prayer requests that are personal to you and your journey in First Place 4 Health. Please complete this form and have it ready to turn in when you arrive at your group meeting.

First Place 4 Health
Prayer Partner

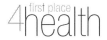

Praise be to the Lord, to God our Savior, who daily bears our burdens.

PSALM 68:19

Date: _____

Name: _____

Home Phone: (_____)_____

Work Phone: (_____)_____

Email: _____

Personal Prayer Concerns:

_____

_____

_____

_____

_____

_____

_____

This form is for prayer requests that are personal to you and your journey in First Place 4 Health. Please complete this form and have it ready to turn in when you arrive at your group meeting.

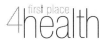
FIT & HEALTHY
SUMMER
Week
3

Blessed are those whose strength is in you, who have set their hearts on pilgrimage.

PSALM 84:5

Date: _____

Name: _____

Home Phone: (_____)_____

Work Phone: (_____)_____

Email: _____

Personal Prayer Concerns:

_____
_____
_____
_____
_____
_____
_____

This form is for prayer requests that are personal to you and your journey in First Place 4 Health. Please complete this form and have it ready to turn in when you arrive at your group meeting.

First Place 4 Health
Prayer Partner

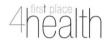

My soul finds rest in God alone; my salvation comes from him.

PSALM 62:1

Date: _____

Name: _____

Home Phone: (_____)_____

Work Phone: (_____)_____

Email: _____

Personal Prayer Concerns:

_____
_____
_____
_____
_____
_____
_____

This form is for prayer requests that are personal to you and your journey in First Place 4 Health. Please complete this form and have it ready to turn in when you arrive at your group meeting.

First Place 4 Health
Prayer Partner

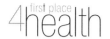

*Though I walk in the midst of trouble, you preserve my life; you stretch out your
hand against the anger of my foes, with your right hand you save me.*

PSALM 138:7

Date: _____

Name: _____

Home Phone: (_____) _____

Work Phone: (_____) _____

Email: _____

Personal Prayer Concerns:

_____

_____

_____

_____

_____

_____

_____

This form is for prayer requests that are personal to you and your journey in First Place 4 Health. Please complete this
form and have it ready to turn in when you arrive at your group meeting.

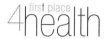

FIT & HEALTHY
SUMMER
Week
6

I am still confident of this: I will see the goodness of the LORD in the land of the living.

PSALM 27:13

Date: _____

Name: _____

Home Phone: (_____) _____

Work Phone: (_____) _____

Email: _____

Personal Prayer Concerns:

_____
_____
_____
_____
_____
_____
_____

This form is for prayer requests that are personal to you and your journey in First Place 4 Health. Please complete this form and have it ready to turn in when you arrive at your group meeting.

Live It Tracker

Name: _____ Loss/gain: _____ lbs.

Date: _____ Week #: _____ Calorie Range: _____ My food goal for next week: _____

Activity Level: None, < 30 min/day, 30-60 min/day, 60+ min/day   My activity goal for next week: _____

Group	Daily Calories							
	1300-1400	1500-1600	1700-1800	1900-2000	2100-2200	2300-2400	2500-2600	2700-2800
Fruits	1.5-2 c.	1.5-2 c.	1.5-2 c.	2-2.5 c.	2-2.5 c.	2.5-3.5 c.	3.5-4.5 c.	3.5-4.5 c.
Vegetables	1.5-2 c.	2-2.5 c.	2.5-3 c.	2.5-3 c.	3-3.5 c.	3.5-4.5 c.	4.5-5 c.	4.5-5 c.
Grains	5 oz-eq.	5-6 oz-eq.	6-7 oz-eq.	6-7 oz-eq.	7-8 oz-eq.	8-9 oz-eq.	9-10 oz-eq.	10-11 oz-eq.
Meat & Beans	4 oz-eq.	5 oz-eq.	5-5.5 oz-eq.	5.5-6.5 oz-eq.	6.5-7 oz-eq.	7-7.5 oz-eq.	7-7.5 oz-eq.	7.5-8 oz-eq.
Milk	2-3 c.	3 c.	3 c.	3 c.	3 c.	3 c.	3 c.	3 c.
Healthy Oils	4 tsp.	5 tsp.	5 tsp.	6 tsp.	6 tsp.	7 tsp.	8 tsp.	8 tsp.

Day/Date: _____

Breakfast: _____   Lunch: _____

Dinner: _____   Snack: _____

Group	Fruits	Vegetables	Grains	Meat & Beans	Milk	Oils
Goal Amount						
Estimate Your Total						
Increase ⇧ or Decrease? ⇩						

Physical Activity: _____   Spiritual Activity: _____

Steps/Miles/Minutes: _____   _____

Day/Date: _____

Breakfast: _____   Lunch: _____

Dinner: _____   Snack: _____

Group	Fruits	Vegetables	Grains	Meat & Beans	Milk	Oils
Goal Amount						
Estimate Your Total						
Increase ⇧ or Decrease? ⇩						

Physical Activity: _____   Spiritual Activity: _____

Steps/Miles/Minutes: _____   _____

Day/Date: _____

Breakfast: _____   Lunch: _____

Dinner: _____   Snack: _____

Group	Fruits	Vegetables	Grains	Meat & Beans	Milk	Oils
Goal Amount						
Estimate Your Total						
Increase ⇧ or Decrease? ⇩						

Physical Activity: _____   Spiritual Activity: _____

Steps/Miles/Minutes: _____   _____

Day/Date:

Breakfast: _____ Lunch: _____

_____

Dinner: _____ Snack: _____

_____

Group	Fruits	Vegetables	Grains	Meat & Beans	Milk	Oils
Goal Amount						
Estimate Your Total						
Increase ⇧ or Decrease? ⇩						

Physical Activity: _____ Spiritual Activity: _____

Steps/Miles/Minutes: _____ _____

Day/Date:

Breakfast: _____ Lunch: _____

_____

Dinner: _____ Snack: _____

_____

Group	Fruits	Vegetables	Grains	Meat & Beans	Milk	Oils
Goal Amount						
Estimate Your Total						
Increase ⇧ or Decrease? ⇩						

Physical Activity: _____ Spiritual Activity: _____

Steps/Miles/Minutes: _____ _____

Day/Date:

Breakfast: _____ Lunch: _____

_____

Dinner: _____ Snack: _____

_____

Group	Fruits	Vegetables	Grains	Meat & Beans	Milk	Oils
Goal Amount						
Estimate Your Total						
Increase ⇧ or Decrease? ⇩						

Physical Activity: _____ Spiritual Activity: _____

Steps/Miles/Minutes: _____ _____

Day/Date:

Breakfast: _____ Lunch: _____

_____

Dinner: _____ Snack: _____

_____

Group	Fruits	Vegetables	Grains	Meat & Beans	Milk	Oils
Goal Amount						
Estimate Your Total						
Increase ⇧ or Decrease? ⇩						

Physical Activity: _____ Spiritual Activity: _____

Steps/Miles/Minutes: _____ _____

Live It Tracker

Name: _____   Loss/gain: _____ lbs.

Date: _____ Week #: _____ Calorie Range: _____ My food goal for next week: _____

Activity Level: None, < 30 min/day, 30-60 min/day, 60+ min/day   My activity goal for next week: _____

Group	Daily Calories							
	1300-1400	1500-1600	1700-1800	1900-2000	2100-2200	2300-2400	2500-2600	2700-2800
Fruits	1.5-2 c.	1.5-2 c.	1.5-2 c.	2-2.5 c.	2-2.5 c.	2.5-3.5 c.	3.5-4.5 c.	3.5-4.5 c.
Vegetables	1.5-2 c.	2-2.5 c.	2.5-3 c.	2.5-3 c.	3-3.5 c.	3.5-4.5 c.	4.5-5 c.	4.5-5 c.
Grains	5 oz-eq.	5-6 oz-eq.	6-7 oz-eq.	6-7 oz-eq.	7-8 oz-eq.	8-9 oz-eq.	9-10 oz-eq.	10-11 oz-eq.
Meat & Beans	4 oz-eq.	5 oz-eq.	5-5.5 oz-eq.	5.5-6.5 oz-eq.	6.5-7 oz-eq.	7-7.5 oz-eq.	7-7.5 oz-eq.	7.5-8 oz-eq.
Milk	2-3 c.	3 c.	3 c.	3 c.	3 c.	3 c.	3 c.	3 c.
Healthy Oils	4 tsp.	5 tsp.	5 tsp.	6 tsp.	6 tsp.	7 tsp.	8 tsp.	8 tsp.

Day/Date:

Breakfast: _____   Lunch: _____

Dinner: _____   Snack: _____

Group	Fruits	Vegetables	Grains	Meat & Beans	Milk	Oils
Goal Amount						
Estimate Your Total						
Increase ⇧ or Decrease? ⇩						

Physical Activity: _____   Spiritual Activity: _____

Steps/Miles/Minutes: _____   _____

Day/Date:

Breakfast: _____   Lunch: _____

Dinner: _____   Snack: _____

Group	Fruits	Vegetables	Grains	Meat & Beans	Milk	Oils
Goal Amount						
Estimate Your Total						
Increase ⇧ or Decrease? ⇩						

Physical Activity: _____   Spiritual Activity: _____

Steps/Miles/Minutes: _____   _____

Day/Date:

Breakfast: _____   Lunch: _____

Dinner: _____   Snack: _____

Group	Fruits	Vegetables	Grains	Meat & Beans	Milk	Oils
Goal Amount						
Estimate Your Total						
Increase ⇧ or Decrease? ⇩						

Physical Activity: _____   Spiritual Activity: _____

Steps/Miles/Minutes: _____   _____

Day/Date: _____

Breakfast: _____ Lunch: _____

Dinner: _____ Snack: _____

Group	Fruits	Vegetables	Grains	Meat & Beans	Milk	Oils
Goal Amount						
Estimate Your Total						
Increase ⇧ or Decrease? ⇩						

Physical Activity: _____ Spiritual Activity: _____

Steps/Miles/Minutes: _____ _____

Day/Date: _____

Breakfast: _____ Lunch: _____

Dinner: _____ Snack: _____

Group	Fruits	Vegetables	Grains	Meat & Beans	Milk	Oils
Goal Amount						
Estimate Your Total						
Increase ⇧ or Decrease? ⇩						

Physical Activity: _____ Spiritual Activity: _____

Steps/Miles/Minutes: _____ _____

Day/Date: _____

Breakfast: _____ Lunch: _____

Dinner: _____ Snack: _____

Group	Fruits	Vegetables	Grains	Meat & Beans	Milk	Oils
Goal Amount						
Estimate Your Total						
Increase ⇧ or Decrease? ⇩						

Physical Activity: _____ Spiritual Activity: _____

Steps/Miles/Minutes: _____ _____

Day/Date: _____

Breakfast: _____ Lunch: _____

Dinner: _____ Snack: _____

Group	Fruits	Vegetables	Grains	Meat & Beans	Milk	Oils
Goal Amount						
Estimate Your Total						
Increase ⇧ or Decrease? ⇩						

Physical Activity: _____ Spiritual Activity: _____

Steps/Miles/Minutes: _____ _____

Live It Tracker

Name: _____ Loss/gain: _____ lbs.

Date: _____ Week #: _____ Calorie Range: _____ My food goal for next week: _____

Activity Level: None, < 30 min/day, 30-60 min/day, 60+ min/day My activity goal for next week: _____

Group	Daily Calories							
	1300-1400	1500-1600	1700-1800	1900-2000	2100-2200	2300-2400	2500-2600	2700-2800
Fruits	1.5-2 c.	1.5-2 c.	1.5-2 c.	2-2.5 c.	2-2.5 c.	2.5-3.5 c.	3.5-4.5 c.	3.5-4.5 c.
Vegetables	1.5-2 c.	2-2.5 c.	2.5-3 c.	2.5-3 c.	3-3.5 c.	3.5-4.5 c.	4.5-5 c.	4.5-5 c.
Grains	5 oz-eq.	5-6 oz-eq.	6-7 oz-eq.	6-7 oz-eq.	7-8 oz-eq.	8-9 oz-eq.	9-10 oz-eq.	10-11 oz-eq.
Meat & Beans	4 oz-eq.	5 oz-eq.	5-5.5 oz-eq.	5.5-6.5 oz-eq.	6.5-7 oz-eq.	7-7.5 oz-eq.	7-7.5 oz-eq.	7.5-8 oz-eq.
Milk	2-3 c.	3 c.	3 c.	3 c.	3 c.	3 c.	3 c.	3 c.
Healthy Oils	4 tsp.	5 tsp.	5 tsp.	6 tsp.	6 tsp.	7 tsp.	8 tsp.	8 tsp.

Day/Date: _____

Breakfast: _____ Lunch: _____

Dinner: _____ Snack: _____

Group	Fruits	Vegetables	Grains	Meat & Beans	Milk	Oils
Goal Amount						
Estimate Your Total						
Increase ⇧ or Decrease? ⇩						

Physical Activity: _____ Spiritual Activity: _____

Steps/Miles/Minutes: _____

Day/Date: _____

Breakfast: _____ Lunch: _____

Dinner: _____ Snack: _____

Group	Fruits	Vegetables	Grains	Meat & Beans	Milk	Oils
Goal Amount						
Estimate Your Total						
Increase ⇧ or Decrease? ⇩						

Physical Activity: _____ Spiritual Activity: _____

Steps/Miles/Minutes: _____

Day/Date: _____

Breakfast: _____ Lunch: _____

Dinner: _____ Snack: _____

Group	Fruits	Vegetables	Grains	Meat & Beans	Milk	Oils
Goal Amount						
Estimate Your Total						
Increase ⇧ or Decrease? ⇩						

Physical Activity: _____ Spiritual Activity: _____

Steps/Miles/Minutes: _____

Day/Date: _____

Breakfast: _____ Lunch: _____

Dinner: _____ Snack: _____

Group	Fruits	Vegetables	Grains	Meat & Beans	Milk	Oils
Goal Amount						
Estimate Your Total						
Increase ⇧ or Decrease? ⇩						

Physical Activity: _____ Spiritual Activity: _____

Steps/Miles/Minutes: _____ _____

Day/Date: _____

Breakfast: _____ Lunch: _____

Dinner: _____ Snack: _____

Group	Fruits	Vegetables	Grains	Meat & Beans	Milk	Oils
Goal Amount						
Estimate Your Total						
Increase ⇧ or Decrease? ⇩						

Physical Activity: _____ Spiritual Activity: _____

Steps/Miles/Minutes: _____ _____

Day/Date: _____

Breakfast: _____ Lunch: _____

Dinner: _____ Snack: _____

Group	Fruits	Vegetables	Grains	Meat & Beans	Milk	Oils
Goal Amount						
Estimate Your Total						
Increase ⇧ or Decrease? ⇩						

Physical Activity: _____ Spiritual Activity: _____

Steps/Miles/Minutes: _____ _____

Day/Date: _____

Breakfast: _____ Lunch: _____

Dinner: _____ Snack: _____

Group	Fruits	Vegetables	Grains	Meat & Beans	Milk	Oils
Goal Amount						
Estimate Your Total						
Increase ⇧ or Decrease? ⇩						

Physical Activity: _____ Spiritual Activity: _____

Steps/Miles/Minutes: _____ _____

Live It Tracker

Name: _____ Loss/gain: _____ lbs.

Date: _____ Week #: _____ Calorie Range: _____ My food goal for next week: _____

Activity Level: None, < 30 min/day, 30-60 min/day, 60+ min/day   My activity goal for next week: _____

Group	Daily Calories							
	1300-1400	1500-1600	1700-1800	1900-2000	2100-2200	2300-2400	2500-2600	2700-2800
Fruits	1.5-2 c.	1.5-2 c.	1.5-2 c.	2-2.5 c.	2-2.5 c.	2.5-3.5 c.	3.5-4.5 c.	3.5-4.5 c.
Vegetables	1.5-2 c.	2-2.5 c.	2.5-3 c.	2.5-3 c.	3-3.5 c.	3.5-4.5 c.	4.5-5 c.	4.5-5 c.
Grains	5 oz-eq.	5-6 oz-eq.	6-7 oz-eq.	6-7 oz-eq.	7-8 oz-eq.	8-9 oz-eq.	9-10 oz-eq.	10-11 oz-eq.
Meat & Beans	4 oz-eq.	5 oz-eq.	5-5.5 oz-eq.	5.5-6.5 oz-eq.	6.5-7 oz-eq.	7-7.5 oz-eq.	7-7.5 oz-eq.	7.5-8 oz-eq.
Milk	2-3 c.	3 c.	3 c.	3 c.	3 c.	3 c.	3 c.	3 c.
Healthy Oils	4 tsp.	5 tsp.	5 tsp.	6 tsp.	6 tsp.	7 tsp.	8 tsp.	8 tsp.

Day/Date:

Breakfast: _____   Lunch: _____

Dinner: _____   Snack: _____

Group	Fruits	Vegetables	Grains	Meat & Beans	Milk	Oils
Goal Amount						
Estimate Your Total						
Increase ⇧ or Decrease? ⇩						

Physical Activity: _____   Spiritual Activity: _____

Steps/Miles/Minutes: _____   _____

Day/Date:

Breakfast: _____   Lunch: _____

Dinner: _____   Snack: _____

Group	Fruits	Vegetables	Grains	Meat & Beans	Milk	Oils
Goal Amount						
Estimate Your Total						
Increase ⇧ or Decrease? ⇩						

Physical Activity: _____   Spiritual Activity: _____

Steps/Miles/Minutes: _____   _____

Day/Date:

Breakfast: _____   Lunch: _____

Dinner: _____   Snack: _____

Group	Fruits	Vegetables	Grains	Meat & Beans	Milk	Oils
Goal Amount						
Estimate Your Total						
Increase ⇧ or Decrease? ⇩						

Physical Activity: _____   Spiritual Activity: _____

Steps/Miles/Minutes: _____   _____

Day/Date: _____

Breakfast: _____ Lunch: _____

Dinner: _____ Snack: _____

Group	Fruits	Vegetables	Grains	Meat & Beans	Milk	Oils
Goal Amount						
Estimate Your Total						
Increase ⇧ or Decrease? ⇩						

Physical Activity: _____ Spiritual Activity: _____

Steps/Miles/Minutes: _____ _____

Day/Date: _____

Breakfast: _____ Lunch: _____

Dinner: _____ Snack: _____

Group	Fruits	Vegetables	Grains	Meat & Beans	Milk	Oils
Goal Amount						
Estimate Your Total						
Increase ⇧ or Decrease? ⇩						

Physical Activity: _____ Spiritual Activity: _____

Steps/Miles/Minutes: _____ _____

Day/Date: _____

Breakfast: _____ Lunch: _____

Dinner: _____ Snack: _____

Group	Fruits	Vegetables	Grains	Meat & Beans	Milk	Oils
Goal Amount						
Estimate Your Total						
Increase ⇧ or Decrease? ⇩						

Physical Activity: _____ Spiritual Activity: _____

Steps/Miles/Minutes: _____ _____

Day/Date: _____

Breakfast: _____ Lunch: _____

Dinner: _____ Snack: _____

Group	Fruits	Vegetables	Grains	Meat & Beans	Milk	Oils
Goal Amount						
Estimate Your Total						
Increase ⇧ or Decrease? ⇩						

Physical Activity: _____ Spiritual Activity: _____

Steps/Miles/Minutes: _____ _____

Live It Tracker

Name: _____ Loss/gain: _____ lbs.

Date: _____ Week #: _____ Calorie Range: _____ My food goal for next week: _____

Activity Level: None, < 30 min/day, 30-60 min/day, 60+ min/day My activity goal for next week: _____

Group	Daily Calories							
	1300-1400	1500-1600	1700-1800	1900-2000	2100-2200	2300-2400	2500-2600	2700-2800
Fruits	1.5-2 c.	1.5-2 c.	1.5-2 c.	2-2.5 c.	2-2.5 c.	2.5-3.5 c.	3.5-4.5 c.	3.5-4.5 c.
Vegetables	1.5-2 c.	2-2.5 c.	2.5-3 c.	2.5-3 c.	3-3.5 c.	3.5-4.5 c.	4.5-5 c.	4.5-5 c.
Grains	5 oz-eq.	5-6 oz-eq.	6-7 oz-eq.	6-7 oz-eq.	7-8 oz-eq.	8-9 oz-eq.	9-10 oz-eq.	10-11 oz-eq.
Meat & Beans	4 oz-eq.	5 oz-eq.	5-5.5 oz-eq.	5.5-6.5 oz-eq.	6.5-7 oz-eq.	7-7.5 oz-eq.	7-7.5 oz-eq.	7.5-8 oz-eq.
Milk	2-3 c.	3 c.	3 c.	3 c.	3 c.	3 c.	3 c.	3 c.
Healthy Oils	4 tsp.	5 tsp.	5 tsp.	6 tsp.	6 tsp.	7 tsp.	8 tsp.	8 tsp.

Day/Date: _____

Breakfast: _____ Lunch: _____

Dinner: _____ Snack: _____

Group	Fruits	Vegetables	Grains	Meat & Beans	Milk	Oils
Goal Amount						
Estimate Your Total						
Increase ⇧ or Decrease? ⇩						

Physical Activity: _____ Spiritual Activity: _____

Steps/Miles/Minutes: _____

Day/Date: _____

Breakfast: _____ Lunch: _____

Dinner: _____ Snack: _____

Group	Fruits	Vegetables	Grains	Meat & Beans	Milk	Oils
Goal Amount						
Estimate Your Total						
Increase ⇧ or Decrease? ⇩						

Physical Activity: _____ Spiritual Activity: _____

Steps/Miles/Minutes: _____

Day/Date: _____

Breakfast: _____ Lunch: _____

Dinner: _____ Snack: _____

Group	Fruits	Vegetables	Grains	Meat & Beans	Milk	Oils
Goal Amount						
Estimate Your Total						
Increase ⇧ or Decrease? ⇩						

Physical Activity: _____ Spiritual Activity: _____

Steps/Miles/Minutes: _____

Day/Date:

Breakfast: _____ Lunch: _____

Dinner: _____ Snack: _____

Group	Fruits	Vegetables	Grains	Meat & Beans	Milk	Oils
Goal Amount						
Estimate Your Total						
Increase ⇧ or Decrease? ⇩						

Physical Activity: _____ Spiritual Activity: _____

Steps/Miles/Minutes: _____ _____

Day/Date:

Breakfast: _____ Lunch: _____

Dinner: _____ Snack: _____

Group	Fruits	Vegetables	Grains	Meat & Beans	Milk	Oils
Goal Amount						
Estimate Your Total						
Increase ⇧ or Decrease? ⇩						

Physical Activity: _____ Spiritual Activity: _____

Steps/Miles/Minutes: _____ _____

Day/Date:

Breakfast: _____ Lunch: _____

Dinner: _____ Snack: _____

Group	Fruits	Vegetables	Grains	Meat & Beans	Milk	Oils
Goal Amount						
Estimate Your Total						
Increase ⇧ or Decrease? ⇩						

Physical Activity: _____ Spiritual Activity: _____

Steps/Miles/Minutes: _____ _____

Day/Date:

Breakfast: _____ Lunch: _____

Dinner: _____ Snack: _____

Group	Fruits	Vegetables	Grains	Meat & Beans	Milk	Oils
Goal Amount						
Estimate Your Total						
Increase ⇧ or Decrease? ⇩						

Physical Activity: _____ Spiritual Activity: _____

Steps/Miles/Minutes: _____ _____

Live It Tracker

Name: _____ Loss/gain: _____ lbs.

Date: _____ Week #: _____ Calorie Range: _____ My food goal for next week: _____

Activity Level: None, < 30 min/day, 30-60 min/day, 60+ min/day My activity goal for next week: _____

Group	Daily Calories							
	1300-1400	1500-1600	1700-1800	1900-2000	2100-2200	2300-2400	2500-2600	2700-2800
Fruits	1.5-2 c.	1.5-2 c.	1.5-2 c.	2-2.5 c.	2-2.5 c.	2.5-3.5 c.	3.5-4.5 c.	3.5-4.5 c.
Vegetables	1.5-2 c.	2-2.5 c.	2.5-3 c.	2.5-3 c.	3-3.5 c.	3.5-4.5 c.	4.5-5 c.	4.5-5 c.
Grains	5 oz-eq.	5-6 oz-eq.	6-7 oz-eq.	6-7 oz-eq.	7-8 oz-eq.	8-9 oz-eq.	9-10 oz-eq.	10-11 oz-eq.
Meat & Beans	4 oz-eq.	5 oz-eq.	5-5.5 oz-eq.	5.5-6.5 oz-eq.	6.5-7 oz-eq.	7-7.5 oz-eq.	7-7.5 oz-eq.	7.5-8 oz-eq.
Milk	2-3 c.	3 c.	3 c.	3 c.	3 c.	3 c.	3 c.	3 c.
Healthy Oils	4 tsp.	5 tsp.	5 tsp.	6 tsp.	6 tsp.	7 tsp.	8 tsp.	8 tsp.

Day/Date:

Breakfast: _____ Lunch: _____

Dinner: _____ Snack: _____

Group	Fruits	Vegetables	Grains	Meat & Beans	Milk	Oils
Goal Amount						
Estimate Your Total						
Increase ⇧ or Decrease? ⇩						

Physical Activity: _____ Spiritual Activity: _____

Steps/Miles/Minutes: _____

Day/Date:

Breakfast: _____ Lunch: _____

Dinner: _____ Snack: _____

Group	Fruits	Vegetables	Grains	Meat & Beans	Milk	Oils
Goal Amount						
Estimate Your Total						
Increase ⇧ or Decrease? ⇩						

Physical Activity: _____ Spiritual Activity: _____

Steps/Miles/Minutes: _____

Day/Date:

Breakfast: _____ Lunch: _____

Dinner: _____ Snack: _____

Group	Fruits	Vegetables	Grains	Meat & Beans	Milk	Oils
Goal Amount						
Estimate Your Total						
Increase ⇧ or Decrease? ⇩						

Physical Activity: _____ Spiritual Activity: _____

Steps/Miles/Minutes: _____

Day/Date: ___

Breakfast: _____   Lunch: _____

Dinner: _____   Snack: _____

Group	Fruits	Vegetables	Grains	Meat & Beans	Milk	Oils
Goal Amount						
Estimate Your Total						
Increase ⇧ or Decrease? ⇩						

Physical Activity: _____   Spiritual Activity: _____

Steps/Miles/Minutes: _____

Day/Date: ___

Breakfast: _____   Lunch: _____

Dinner: _____   Snack: _____

Group	Fruits	Vegetables	Grains	Meat & Beans	Milk	Oils
Goal Amount						
Estimate Your Total						
Increase ⇧ or Decrease? ⇩						

Physical Activity: _____   Spiritual Activity: _____

Steps/Miles/Minutes: _____

Day/Date: ___

Breakfast: _____   Lunch: _____

Dinner: _____   Snack: _____

Group	Fruits	Vegetables	Grains	Meat & Beans	Milk	Oils
Goal Amount						
Estimate Your Total						
Increase ⇧ or Decrease? ⇩						

Physical Activity: _____   Spiritual Activity: _____

Steps/Miles/Minutes: _____

Day/Date: ___

Breakfast: _____   Lunch: _____

Dinner: _____   Snack: _____

Group	Fruits	Vegetables	Grains	Meat & Beans	Milk	Oils
Goal Amount						
Estimate Your Total						
Increase ⇧ or Decrease? ⇩						

Physical Activity: _____   Spiritual Activity: _____

Steps/Miles/Minutes: _____